DELUSIONAL DISORDER
Paranoia and Related Illnesses

Delusional disorder, once termed paranoia, was an important diagnosis in the late nineteenth and early twentieth centuries. Subsequently it was subsumed with schizophrenia, and only in 1987 was it reintroduced into modern psychiatric diagnosis. This book aims to reconcile recent knowledge with older ideas about the condition, and thereby to provide a contemporary perspective to the concept of delusional disorder and to integrate the scattered literature on the topic.

The illness has a characteristic form, but the content of the delusional system can vary widely. Sufferers may deny mental illness and refuse psychiatric help, so that mental health professionals, who should be at the forefront in dealing with delusional disorder, are often the last to see it. Psychiatrists and other clinicians will therefore appreciate this review of a disorder once considered untreatable but in fact, as the author shows, responsive to appropriate management. The text deals with the emergence of the concept of delusional disorder, and goes on to detail its manifold presentations, differential diagnosis and treatment. Many instructive case histories are provided, illustrating manifestations of delusional disorder including the persecutory and somatic subtypes, and variants including dysmorphic and infestation delusion, erotomania, and related conditions in the paranoid spectrum such as paraphrenia, *folie à deux* and paranoid personality disorder.

This is the most wide ranging and authoritative text on the subject to have appeared for many years, and the first to suggest, based on the author's extensive experience, that the category of delusional disorder should contain not one but several conditions. It also emphasizes that, contrary to traditional belief, delusional disorder is a treatable illness.

ALISTAIR MUNRO is Professor Emeritus of Psychiatry at Dalhousie University, Halifax, Nova Scotia, and an internationally recognized authority on delusional disorder.

Publisher's Note

The Publishers acknowledge their debt to the late George Winokur, MD, who, in the last years of his life, worked with them to develop this book, and three further volumes, as the first titles in a new series under his editorship, to be called *Concepts in Clinical Psychiatry*. Dr Winokur was not, unfortunately, able to read any of these works in their final form.

Dr Winokur's contribution to contemporary psychiatry, and in particular his dedication to a medical model for psychiatric disorder, was distinctive, and his editorial style was inimitable. These four volumes are a tribute to his vision for psychiatry as a clinical discipline founded on the principles of scientific evidence and clinical judgement.

The Anxiety Disorders
by Russell Noyes, Jr., and Rudolf Hoehn-Saric

Delusional Disorder
Paranoia and related illnesses
by Alistair Munro

Schizophrenia
Concepts and clinical management
by Eve C. Johnstone, Martin Humphreys, Fiona Lang, Stephen Lawrie and Robert Sandler

Somatoform and Dissociative Disorders
by William R. Yates, Carol S. North and Richard D. Wetzel

DELUSIONAL DISORDER

Paranoia and Related Illnesses

ALISTAIR MUNRO
Dalhousie University, Halifax, Nova Scotia

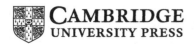

CAMBRIDGE
UNIVERSITY PRESS

CAMBRIDGE UNIVERSITY PRESS
Cambridge, New York, Melbourne, Madrid, Cape Town, Singapore, São Paulo

Cambridge University Press
The Edinburgh Building, Cambridge CB2 2RU, UK

Published in the United States of America by Cambridge University Press, New York

www.cambridge.org
Information on this title: www.cambridge.org/9780521581806

First published 1999
This digitally printed first paperback version 2006

A catalogue record for this publication is available from the British Library

Library of Congress Cataloguing in Publication data
Munro, Alistair.
Delusional disorder: paranoia and related illnesses/Alistair Munro.
   p.   cm.
1. Delusions.   2. Delusions–case studies.   3. Paranoia.
I. Title.
RC553.D35M86   1998
616.89′7–dc21   98–17210 CIP

ISBN-13 978-0-521-58180-6 hardback
ISBN-10 0-521-58180-X hardback

ISBN-13 978-0-521-02980-3 paperback
ISBN-10 0-521-02980-5 paperback

Every effort has been made in preparing this publication to provide accurate and up-to-date
information which is in accord with accepted standards and practice at the time of
publication. Nevertheless, the authors, editors and publisher can make no warranties that
the information contained herein is totally free from error, not least because clinical
standards are constantly changing through research and regulation. The authors, editors
and publisher therefore disclaim all liability for direct or consequential damages resulting
from the use of material contained in this publication. Readers are strongly advised to pay
careful attention to information provided by the manufacturer of any drugs or equipment that
they plan to use.

To my wife Mary, who 'not only tolerated, but encouraged'

Contents

Case descriptions

Preface

Paranoia and its related disorders were regarded as an important group of psychiatric illnesses until the early part of the twentieth century. Then, because of prevalent classification practices – particularly the tendency to overdiagnose schizophrenia – the diagnoses of paranoia and paraphrenia virtually died out. In 1987, paranoia was revived by DSMIIIR and was renamed 'delusional disorder': as such, it currently is the only officially recognized member of the old paranoid disorder clustering.

Although the diagnosis disappeared, the illness and its sufferers did not. The result was both an inappropriate 'lumping' of cases of delusional disorder into other categories, most usually schizophrenia, and an extraordinary 'splitting', in which cases of paranoia/delusional disorders were recognized for some secondary feature, but their true diagnosis was ignored. The latter especially has meant a profoundly scattered literature and a great deal of confusion as to what is delusional illness and what is not.

This book is an attempt to define more clearly the concept of paranoia/ delusional disorder and to gather the shards of the current body of knowledge into a more coherent whole. It also tries to define the limits of delusional disorders and to dispel some of the confusion which still exists when trying to exclude vaguely similar illnesses. At the same time, a strong effort is made to point out that paranoia/delusional disorder is not the only 'delusional disorder': for example, paraphrenia and delusional misidentification syndromes (DMS) are strong candidates for inclusion in an expanded category.

Although written primarily for psychiatrists, this volume should be of considerable interest to many other specialties and professions. For example, general physicians, plastic surgeons, dermatologists and gastroenterologists, among others, all become involved with individuals who have somatic delusions, and neurologists increasingly see cases of DMS.

Lawyers and law enforcement personnel are frequently involved with individuals who offend because of jealous or erotomanic delusions and who may stalk or assault their victims. Social workers and others in the community field deal with many deluded clients, and even pest control officers have an interest since they are not infrequently called in to disinfest houses by individuals who believe they are assailed by parasitic organisms.

The contents of the book are technical but, so far as possible, the style has been kept jargon-free and eschews unnecessary speculation. It is designed to be a practical guide to professionals, whether medical or not, who are curious about these fascinating illnesses and who may require some apposite and up-to-date knowledge to recognize and deal with them in their particular settings. Frequent case-examples are provided to emphasize what are, and what are not, features of the various subtypes.

Throughout the book, unless the sex of an individual is specifically indicated, the words 'he' and 'she' should be regarded as interchangeable.

I wish to express my gratitude to Sharon C. Munro, Reference/Collections Librarian, Leddy Library, the University of Windsor, Ontario, Canada for her great help in tracing the less accessible references I needed for this book. I would also like to thank Mr. Robert Lennie for his considered comments on the contents of the manuscript, and Marilyn Harper for its meticulous preparation.

As always, my particular thanks go to my wife and family for their tolerance while I struggled (not always amiably) with this project.

Unless otherwise stated, all literary quotations throughout the book are taken from *Bartlett's Familiar Quotations*, 15th edition, published in 1980 by Little, Brown and Co.

A.M.

Part I
Delusional disorders and delusions: introductory aspects

He who would distinguish the true from the false must have an adequate idea of what is true and false.
Benedict Spinoza (1632–1677)

Delusional disorder, under its former soubriquet of paranoia, is a venerable diagnosis. Unfortunately both the concept and the diagnosis fell into abeyance in the early part of the twentieth century and have only come back into prominence since 1987, when paranoia – renamed delusional disorder – was revived in DSMIIIR (the revised third edition of the American Psychiatric Association's *Diagnostic and Statistical Manual of Mental Disorders*). It has subsequently been confirmed in the tenth revision of the World Health Association's *International Statistical Classification of Diseases* (ICD10, 1992–93) and in DSMIV (1994) and, as will unfold in the course of this book, a considerable world-wide and cross-disciplinary literature on the subject has grown up in recent years.

To many mental health professionals, delusional disorder remains a shadowy concept and it is quite possible for a psychiatrist to have a busy practice and either not see, or not recognize, cases of the illness. This arises from a combination of lack of knowledge about it and of relative rarity in the psychiatrist's office of patients with the disorder: the reasons for the latter will be explored later.

In this section, an introduction to the disorder is undertaken and we will consider why the disorder appears to have such an elusive quality. A cursory knowledge of the evolution of paranoia/delusional disorder is essential as a background to the consideration of this elusiveness and, as will become apparent, this process has been extraordinarily complex and its sources extremely fragmented.

Finally, we shall consider briefly several aspects of the phenomena associated with delusions, the principal feature on which the diagnosis of delusional disorder depends. Here, the literature is much more coherent but it will emerge that many of our preconceptions about delusions are highly debatable and that even the best experimental work in the field may not always translate into applications which are useful in the clinical field.

1

Outline and introduction: a brief perspective on the delusional disorders

This chapter will be divided into three sections: (*a*) an introduction to the delusional disorders; (*b*) a concise description of the derivation of current concepts regarding delusional disorders; and (*c*) some notes on phenomena associated with delusions.

An introduction to the delusional disorders

Delusional disorder is an accepted diagnosis nowadays but many aspects of its description still stem from writings of the late nineteenth and early twentieth centuries, and modern descriptions are still only a few years old.

In writing about paranoia/delusional disorder (these terms will be discussed in detail later) there are two misconceptions which must be countered. The first is that it is rare. Certainly, cases do not appear in profusion in the average psychiatrist's office but, as will be shown in Chapters 2 and 3, there are many references to different manifestations of the illness in several literatures, of which the psychiatric is but one. Cumulatively, these create an impression of a disorder that is far from unusual. In addition, because many cases remain unrecognized in the community (see p.51) it is possible that delusional disorder in its various degrees of severity is really quite common. But this is guesswork and all that we are justified in saying at present is that it is not nearly so rare as psychiatrists believe and that, rather oddly, psychiatrists are often the last professional people to see such cases.

The second misconception is that the illness is untreatable. It is not so long ago that virtually all psychiatric disorders were inaccessible to therapy, but we take it for granted now that many of them respond to treatment, whether it is pharmacological or psychological or, very often, a combination of both. As will be described, delusional disorder as a distinct diagnosis faded from view at a time of therapeutic hopelessness in psychiatry and only returned to our awareness in the 1970s and 1980s.

For many physicians not familiar with the modern literature, the illness is still saddled with an extremely gloomy outlook. In fact, Chapter 13 underlines the new attitude of optimism we can adopt with an illness which, if allowed to go untreated, is certainly both severe and disabling, but which, adequately treated, may have one of the more hopeful prognoses of the severe psychiatric disorders.

A note on terminology

In the late nineteenth century the paranoid illnesses were a well-recognized group of disorders and, of these, paranoia was the most notable with the addition, in the early twentieth century, of paraphrenia as a relatively close second. Thereafter, as will be described, these terms increasingly lost favour while paranoid schizophrenia and paranoid personality disorder became well-established diagnostic concepts.

As well as this, 'paranoia' and 'paranoid' became common laymen's terms, usually implying habitual attitudes of distrust, suspiciousness and irritability in an individual rather than any specific psychiatric illness.

With the appearance of the American Psychiatric Association's *Diagnostic and Statistical Manual of Mental Disorders*, third edition, revised (DSMIIIR) in 1987, paranoia was revived as a distinct disorder but was renamed 'delusional (paranoid) disorder' and given its own separate category. Currently, the term 'delusional disorder' represents both a category of psychiatric illness and the only disorder which that category subsumes. Subtypes of delusional disorder are distinguished by the predominant content of the delusional system, for example persecutory, grandiose, somatic, etc. Paraphrenia at this time has no recognized diagnostic status in our official diagnostic systems, but a case will be made later in the book for its reinstatement.

In the 1970s, the present author wrote extensively on a delusional illness characterized by somatic complaints and referred to at the time as 'monosymptomatic hypochondriacal psychosis' (or MHP), a name derived from the German and Scandinavian psychiatric literatures. It has since become apparent that this is a subtype of delusional disorder, as now described in the *Diagnostic and Statistical Manual of Mental Disorders*, fourth edition (DSMIV) and in the *International Statistical Classification of Diseases*, tenth edition (ICD10), and in recent years it has seemed best to give up the use of the term 'monosymptomatic hypochondriacal psychosis' and refer instead to 'delusional disorder, somatic subtype'.

In the present volume, paranoia and delusional disorder are regarded as one and the same thing and the names are used synonymously or, at times, in conjunction as 'paranoia/delusional disorder' to underline that synonymity. As has been explained above, 'delusional disorder, somatic subtype' and 'monosymptomatic hypochondriacal psychosis' are also interchangeable with each other, but the former will invariably be used except to make some special point. Both DSMIV and ICD10 utilize the term 'delusional disorder' and it has rapidly gained precedence over older terminologies: it makes good sense, therefore, to employ it preferentially and to refer to its different subtypes to ensure uniformity. Where older terms are introduced from time to time, an attempt will always be made to explain how these relate to modern usages.

However, conventional classifications and jargon are rarely infallible and an argument will be put forward for necessary changes to the current views of DSMIV and ICD10 on delusional disorders.

For a variety of reasons which will be considered later, the concept of paranoia had 'fallen into abatement and low price' by the mid-twentieth century. It had gradually come to be described in the textbooks in the most perfunctory way, if it was mentioned at all. Indeed, one standard British text of the time went so far as to say it probably did not exist at all (Mayer-Gross, Slater and Roth, 1960).

Now that paranoia has returned to respectability under its new title of delusional disorder, however, and cases are being recognized with increasing commonness, does it not seem odd that a whole illness category could simply vanish for several decades? In Chapter 2 this situation will be examined in rather more detail with an attempt to explain how it could happen.

Of course, it is obvious that the cases did not disappear. Instead they were viewed differently and were usually placed under the (then) catch-all rubric of schizophrenia. Because paranoia really does not resemble schizophrenia very closely, cases would be diagnosed as aberrant forms of the latter: but schizophrenia was seen as having so many aberrant presentations that another one seemed to make little difference. For many years, therefore, psychiatrists of this author's generation saw cases of paranoia but did not have the knowledge to appreciate that this was an illness in its own right.

The recognition of cases of delusional disorder

There has been a considerable renaissance regarding paranoia/delusional disorder since the early 1980s, at first concentrating to a considerable extent on the somatic subtype (i.e. MHP) but latterly looking at the other subtypes and at the illness in general. Unfortunately, much of the current literature is anecdotal and based on a large number of very small case samples, and it is scattered across many journals in several disciplines. There is a growing number of knowledgeable contributors in the area but the awareness of delusional disorder among psychiatrists in general is still somewhat restricted. This is one reason why the present volume has been written, as an attempt to gather together some very disparate material, to provide an overview, and to inform clinicians about an important, though still imperfectly appreciated, psychiatric disorder.

Another factor as to why delusional disorders still sometimes seem obscure is that many of their sufferers continue to be quite high-functioning and survive to a greater or lesser degree in the community. Also, as part of their delusional belief system they flatly reject any suggestion that they are mentally ill, so they deliberately and often angrily avoid being referred to psychiatrists. This means that many mental health specialists are still unfamiliar with such cases and remain uncomfortable in making a diagnosis. Psychiatric consultants still see too many individuals with delusional disorder wrongly labelled schizoaffective, called an atypical psychosis or given a similar nondescript label. At least we much less often lump the cases with schizophrenia, but psychiatrists and others in the mental health realm still have much to learn about modern concepts of delusional disorder and about how to treat these patients.

Paranoia does not have a good reputation, being associated in most people's minds with anger, suspiciousness, ideas of reference, accusations of persecution and rejection of psychiatric help. These are certainly features of many cases and may make it difficult to engage the individual in treatment. On the other hand, many patients who are viewed as 'paranoid' are actually suffering from severe personality disorder or paranoid schizophrenia and in some ways these are perhaps even more difficult to engage in therapy.

Many anecdotal treatment results, and a small number of double-blind drug trials, appear to show a consensus that delusional disorder, despite its traditional resistance to treatment, can now be regarded as an eminently treatable illness. Munro and Mok (1995) reviewed the world literature (much of which is regrettably incomplete) and found that pimozide tends to be the most widely used drug in different forms of delusional disorder and that it appears to give very good results, but it is pointed out that the evidence is still insufficient to know whether it is inherently superior to other neuroleptics in treating delusional disorder. What is most important, however, is not to urge a particular treatment but rather to underline the treatability of the illness.

The gap of nearly 60 years between the disappearance of paranoia and its reappearance as delusional disorder is a dreadful indictment of the diagnostic standards of the mid-twentieth century. How could we ever have confused paranoia with schizophrenia? Yet we did and, as will be pointed out later, we are still apparently making similar errors in relation to other diagnoses.

This book will attempt to describe the clinical aspects of delusional disorder in an understandable way (using case descriptions as illustrations), to look at delusional disorders in their wider nosological context and, finally, to suggest some ideas for the future. As new investigative methods become available to the clinical neurosciences, that future promises to be an extremely fruitful one; it will be even more fruitful if our diagnostic practices can become more precise *now*, thereby permitting research to concentrate on increasingly homogeneous illness categories.

If the reader is an experienced clinician, the present volume should provide him or her with useful information to help with the more refined diagnosis and treatment of the delusional disorders which occur in his or her clinical work. If, on the other hand, the reader is unfamiliar with the delusional disorders, perhaps what has been written will provide the knowledge that allows for ready recognition when the first case comes along. Nowadays we have much readier access to the older literature as well as to the rapidly growing number of new publications on delusional disorder. We are therefore no longer mapping almost totally unfamiliar territory as was the case only 20 years ago.

Until now, work on delusional disorder has remained largely at the descriptive level and very little that is experimental has as yet emerged. That is a great pity, because it is a condition which could very well reward scientific study. It has certain features which suggest that it may be the outcome of quite circumscribed brain pathology: not least among these suggestions is the rapid return to relatively normal mental function in patients who respond well to a neuroleptic, even when the illness has been of very long duration.

Neurobiological research on this illness might well give us profound insights into important aspects of the psychopathology of psychotic illnesses and of their brain correlates. In addition, since effective treatment is available, we are potentially able to follow the disorder from the wholly untreated to the fully treated stage, making observations each step of the way.

Delusional disorder or disorders?

There is a grey area between the important groupings of the major mood disorders and 'the schizophrenias' (schizophrenia being not a single illness but – more likely – a conglomerate of related disorders). Paranoia/delusional disorder partly fills this in and has some overlap of clinical features with both types of illness. But there are other illnesses in this ill-defined area, not all of them officially recognized by DSMIV and ICD10.

It will be contended that paraphrenia is the most notable of these 'unofficial' disorders, but there are some more which have a more or less accepted existence, and these include cycloid psychosis, brief reactive psychosis (brief psychotic episode) and the delusional misidentification syndromes. Later, an argument will be put forward for the inclusion of paraphrenia in a 'paranoid spectrum' and as a worthy candidate to be a second delusional disorder. Cycloid psychosis and brief psychotic episode are often confused with each other and with delusional disorder, and it has been found necessary to try to disentangle a confusing literature on both in order to clarify their respective features and to demonstrate that each differs markedly from delusional disorder, while being part of its differential diagnosis.

The delusional misidentification syndromes share some important features in common with paranoia/delusional disorder and, on that ground alone, may qualify to be regarded as a further 'delusional disorder'. In addition, fascinating evidence about specific brain abnormalities in these syndromes is accruing and throws potential light on the aetiology of delusional disorder itself. This has been considered in some detail in Chapter 9.

It may seem to some purists that it is inappropriate to give space to these various disorders in a book on delusional disorder, but the literature on delusional disorder has been, until recently, unhelpful in separating it from other illnesses, including schizophrenia, paraphrenia and the other conditions just mentioned. We must be more conversant with all of these in order to be sure when we are, or are not, dealing with a case of delusional disorder *per se*.

The derivation of current concepts regarding delusional disorders

While discussing schizophrenia, Stengel (1957) said, 'There are many indications that differences of theoretical concepts, however vaguely held, are frequently responsible for diagnostic disagreements'. His observation could apply equally to the paranoid/delusional disorders, where psychiatrists have often diagnosed according to preconceived belief rather than by unbiased observation. The career of the paranoid/delusional disorders since the death of Kraepelin is a sad commentary on psychiatry's unhappy tradition of confusing hypothesis with explanation, and its all-too-frequent lack of respect for scientific methodology.

At present, DSMIV (1994) and the international statistical classification of diseases, tenth edition (ICD10) describe only one delusional disorder. In 1981, Kendler and Tsuang, citing respectable authority, listed four illnesses in this category, as follows:

(1) Paranoid schizophrenia.
(2) Paranoid state (which approximates to paraphrenia).
(3) Paranoia (now known as delusional disorder).
(4) Paranoid psychoses of late life (often called 'late paraphrenia').

They excluded paranoid personality disorder since it is not a psychotic condition and it is not associated with delusions. Elsewhere in this book (see Chapter 12) this disorder will be mentioned briefly, mainly to emphasize that differentiation.

Paranoid schizophrenia is not usually included with the paranoid/delusional disorders, though Emil Kraepelin (1909–1913) thought that there were good arguments why it might be. Although this section deals mostly with paranoia and paraphrenia, later in this chapter and elsewhere, some background information on paranoid schizophrenia, late paraphrenia, late onset schizophrenia, brief reactive psychosis, cycloid psychosis, and delusional misidentification syndromes will also be presented, since these illnesses hover uncertainly on the edge of the paranoid/delusional group.

Problems concerning nomenclature

The delusional disorders have often been overshadowed by schizophrenia and, at times, by the mood disorders. The borderlines are admittedly shadowy, yet paranoid/delusional disorders were quite well defined nearly a century ago. Unfortunately, terminology has been a major stumbling block and words like 'paranoia', 'paraphrenia' and 'paranoid' have been used so loosely that even professionals find difficulty in defining them satisfactorily. This situation still gives rise to major problems in discussing this group of illnesses.

Fish (1974) noted that English-speaking psychiatrists customarily use 'paranoid' to mean 'persecutory', whereas strictly speaking it should mean

'delusional'. Kendler and Tsuang (1981) emphasized the need for definitions, as well as inclusion/exclusion criteria for paranoid/delusional disorder, but careful use of definitions concerning these illnesses is still the
exception rather than the rule, although DSMIV and ICD10 certainly
have taken several steps in the right direction.

We speak about paranoid disorders but specifically exclude paranoid
personality disorder. When we talk about paranoid personality disorder
we have to say, 'This is not a paranoid (i.e. delusional) condition'. This is
confusing and logic suggests that, as a minimum, the personality disorder
be given a new name. However, in the preparation of DSMIIIR (1987) it
was considered that psychiatrists would be particularly reluctant to give
up the term, 'paranoid personality disorder'. So, instead, 'paranoid disorders' lost their name and became 'delusional (paranoid) disorders' in
DSMIIIR.

DSMIIIR was very restrictive and DSMIV and ICD10 have remained
so; therefore this new category contains only one disorder, which corresponds largely to the traditional definition of paranoia. Like Kendler and
Tsuang (1981), the present author firmly believes there are several delusional disorders, and it is hoped that new interest in this area will lead to
recognition of some or all of them and provide adequate up-to-date
descriptions of them.

Paranoia until the late nineteenth century

Kraepelin (whom we shall soon mention in more detail) was just beginning
his pioneering work on the reformation of psychiatric classification at this
time and paranoia was only one of many diagnoses whose description
varied widely from one centre to another. Nevertheless, based on the
descriptions already extant in the 1890s, a psychiatrist of that time might
have been able to say the following about paranoia:

(1) It is a stable disorder characterized by the presence of delusions.
(2) It is a primary disorder, not secondary to another psychiatric diag-
    nosis.
(3) It is a chronic disorder: in many cases it appears to persist unaltered
    until death.
(4) The delusions are logically constructed and are internally consistent.
(5) The disorder is a monomania: that is, the delusions have a single and
    consistent theme.
(6) Despite the monodelusional quality, different patients' illnesses have

differing contents, including ideas of influence, persecution and grandiosity.

(7) The individual experiences an exaggerated sense of self-reference.

(8) It is apparently a disorder of the highest aspects of the intellect and,
although affective symptoms may be present, paranoia is not secondary to depressed mood.

(9) Hallucinations can occur, and in some cases may exacerbate the
delusional ideas.

(10) The presence of delusions does not interfere with the individual's
general logical reasoning (although within the delusional system
the logic is perverted) and there is no general disturbance of behaviour.

(11) Many cases appear to arise in the setting of a markedly abnormal
personality.

(12) The frequency of the illness is unknown but it occurs often enough to
make it of some note.

(13) There are many theories of causation, but the aetiology of the disorder is in dispute.

As will be seen in Chapter 2, this is not at all a bad description of
paranoia as perceived at the present time, but unfortunately in 1890 the
situation was like a jigsaw puzzle with many psychiatrists holding separate
pieces, and with no-one quite able to see the overall picture.

It was left to Emil Kraepelin to articulate the principles which go to
make up not only paranoia, but the paranoid/delusional disorders in
general, and to make some kind of coherent construct out of them.

The influence of Kraepelin

Emil Kraepelin is widely considered to be the originator of modern classificatory methods in psychiatry. Following the example of Kahlbaum (1863)
he studied illnesses not only according to their appearances at a given time,
but also according to their characteristic courses over periods of time. His
work on schizophrenia, manic–depressive illness and paranoid/delusional
disorders remains seminal. His famous textbook (*Psychiatrie, Ein Lehrbuch für Studierende und Ärtze*) first appeared in 1883 and eventually ran
to nine editions. It has had an enormous influence on psychiatry, and many
of his views are still widely respected today.

In the 1896 edition of the *Lehrbuch* he described three apparently
separate disorders, dementia praecox (a term he inherited from earlier

workers), catatonia and dementia paranoides, whose ultimate courses appeared to be mental degeneration. He regarded paranoia as a distinct condition with its own course and outcome.

In the next edition (1899) he revised his views on dementia praecox, catatonia and dementia paranoides and proposed that they were different aspects of one illness, to which he gave the overall label, 'dementia praecox', the illness Bleuler (1950) later called 'schizophrenia'. Dementia paranoides included those cases which appeared to meet the criteria of paranoia, except that they thereafter deteriorated rapidly. Paranoia continued to be seen as a separate illness with well-systematized delusions which were not bizarre, with a chronic but nondegenerative course, and with relatively slight involvement of affect and volition.

From then until his death in 1926, Kraepelin maintained his general view of paranoia, although he gradually introduced detailed modifications. Because of opposition from some quarters, he doubted its validity at times and on occasion he considered dropping the diagnosis, but always found it too useful to do so.

He differentiated paranoia distinctly from dementia praecox at all times by insisting that delusions in paranoia were systematized and relatively consistent, nonbizarre, and often related – though pathologically – to real-life events. He believed that persecutory delusions were the most common, followed by delusions of jealousy, grandeur and eroticism. Nowadays, hypochondriacal delusions are also well recognized: Kraepelin observed such delusions but never himself saw a case which he felt was characterized by them. At first, he allowed auditory hallucinations and auditory misinterpretations to be included in the description of paranoia, but in the eighth edition of his textbook (1909–1913) he specifically excluded these.

According to Kraepelin, patients with paranoia had no disturbance of the form of thought, as opposed to the abnormal (delusional) content, and the main defect was considered to be in their judgment. The personality was well-preserved, even though the illness might last several decades and the only behavioural changes were those related to the delusional beliefs. For example, an individual who felt he was persecuted might attack his 'persecutor' but would behave acceptably in every other circumstance. This was in marked distinction to the generally disturbed behaviour of the schizophrenic.

The mood in paranoia can be fairly normal when the patient is not thinking about his delusional ideas, but becomes very intense when he is preoccupied with them. Nevertheless, the mood essentially remains appropriate to the delusional content, and Kraepelin steadfastly maintained that paranoia was not secondary to a disorder of mood.

The illness he described was largely one of middle and older age, the most common onset being between 30 and 40. In his series (of only 19 cases) men outnumbered women. In his description he emphasized that the premorbid personality was frequently abnormal, with lifelong eccentricities and strange attitudes in more than half of his cases. He believed these features caused stresses, setting up a vicious circle which helped to precipitate the illness.

For many years he considered paranoia to be invariably unremitting and incurable. However, in his textbook's eighth edition he did allow for a better prognosis in some cases. While still believing that most cases were unrelenting, he said that milder cases might develop their delusions temporarily as a result of stress and that some of these might be related to manic–depressive illness. In these 'reactive' cases he believed that the paranoia was 'understandable' (see p.15) as an outcome of interaction between environmental stress and a predisposed personality: otherwise he regarded paranoia as an 'endogenous' illness. It is possible that 'reactive' paranoia is the condition now known as 'brief psychotic disorder' (DSMIV) or 'acute and transient psychotic disorder' (ICD), which is described in Chapter 11.

Kraepelin's views on paraphrenia

In the eighth edition of his textbook, Kraepelin introduced a new diagnosis, that of paraphrenia. He described paraphrenia as similar to paranoid schizophrenia, having fantastic delusions and hallucinations, but with relatively slight thought disorder and much better preservation of affect. Compared with schizophrenia, personality deterioration was considerably less and there was little loss of volition. The behaviour of paraphrenic patients was much less disturbed than that of schizophrenics, and even when their delusions were severe they appeared reasonable in manner. Their ability to communicate and to convey affective warmth remained good.

Now that he had described paraphrenia as an illness lying between paranoid schizophrenia and paranoia, Kraepelin was encouraged to say that paranoia did not have hallucinations. So, henceforth a paranoia-like illness with hallucinations would be considered to be paraphrenia. As will be indicated later, this is perhaps the only serious diagnostic mis-step made by Kraepelin in the whole area of paranoid/delusional disorders.

Kraepelin's views on paranoid schizophrenia

While he was defining paranoia and paraphrenia, Kraepelin was pursuing his major task of refining his other diagnoses, especially dementia praecox and manic-depressive insanity.

As has been already noted, he introduced the term 'dementia paranoides' in 1896 to describe a small group of patients with profound and bizarre persecutory and grandiose delusions who showed fairly rapid personality deterioration, marked thought disorder and severe affective symptoms.

As also previously described, in 1899 (op cit) he began to employ 'dementia praecox' to describe much of what is now called schizophrenia, distinguishing three subtypes: hebephrenic, catatonic and paranoid. (Bleuler later added a fourth: simple schizophrenia.) In the paranoid variety he included the severely disturbed dementia paranoides cases as well as patients whose delusions were more systematized and stable and whose general deterioration was slower. In 1903–04, in the textbook's seventh edition, he mentioned that some of the latter did not deteriorate severely at all and did not have the profound incoherence and mood disturbance typical of dementia praecox; some of these cases were later transferred to the paraphrenia category.

His core group of paranoid schizophrenics is essentially the one we recognize today. Their illness comes on relatively late, they deteriorate less than other schizophrenics, but they still show features characteristic of schizophrenia, with generalised thought disorder, affective involvement, and disorder of volition as well as florid delusions and hallucinations.

Other contributions to the conceptualization of the delusional disorders

In 1911, Eugen Bleuler (1857–1939) introduced the term 'schizophrenia' to avoid the twin misconceptions inherent in the name 'dementia praecox', that it was necessarily a deteriorative illness and that it could only occur in the young (Bleuler, 1950). As Kendler and Tsuang (1981) note, Bleuler gave more latitude than Kraepelin in the diagnosis of schizophrenia and he included many of the paranoid illnesses in this category. Nevertheless, he did recognize paranoia as a separate disorder and, in fact, allowed the presence of hallucinations in the diagnosis. At first he recognized paraphrenia but subsequently saw it as a variant of paranoid schizophrenia. In general, his influence led to an over-recognition of schizophrenia for many years, especially in the United States.

Karl Jaspers (1883–1969) struggled to differentiate symptoms such as delusions which were the result of a 'psychic process', a hypothetical mechanism to explain enduring psychological symptoms which could not be 'understood' from other symptoms which could be recognized as a 'development' from the previous personality. In his concept of 'Verstehende' psychology, schizophrenic symptoms were not understandable, in contrast to many paranoid symptoms which could be comprehended as an outcome of environmental stress impinging on an abnormal personality. His views have been very influential although they continue to generate debate (Huber, 1992), but in our context at least they did seem to support Kraepelin's contention that schizophrenia and paranoid disorders were separate, and also emphasized the frequency of premorbid personality abnormalities in paranoid/delusional disorders.

Ernst Kretschmer (1888–1964) suggested that paranoid symptoms tended to occur in abnormally sensitive individuals who experienced life-long conflict between strong feelings of inadequacy and an unrequited sense of self-importance (Kretschmer, 1927). Under the influence of a 'key experience', an 'understandable' psychosis emerges, with delusions of reference and persecution. Fish (1974) believed that this might explain some delusional contents, but failed to elucidate the paranoid mechanism.

Psychoanalysts believe that the contribution of Sigmund Freud (1856–1939) to the understanding of the paranoid/delusional disorders is basic. Certainly, his descriptions (1958a, b) of the putative mental mechanisms involved in paranoia are useful as metaphors, but his diagnostic approach was loose and his nomenclatures confusing. However, he did say that paranoia and dementia praecox should be seen as distinct disorders.

While the Kraepelinian view of paranoid disorder has proved the most enduring one, it has not necessarily been accepted everywhere. As Fish pointed out, many European psychiatrists did not accept paranoid disorders as separate illnesses but instead regarded paranoid conditions as expressions of other mental illnesses such as schizophrenia, affective disorder, organic brain disorder or as psychogenic reactions secondary to environmental stress acting upon an abnormal personality. It should be appreciated that this viewpoint is still prevalent in parts of Europe (Berner, 1965; Retterstøl, 1966), and is radically different from present-day practice in the English-speaking world. In DSMIV and ICD10, delusional disorder is essentially and specifically Kraepelinian paranoia and not a group of illnesses.

Subsequent developments

Paranoia

In 1931, after Kraepelin's death, Kolle reported his study of primary paranoia, describing the detailed follow-up of 66 cases seen in Kraepelin's former clinic in Munich. Despite the fact that a proportion of the cases of paranoia retained these original features, he emphasized those which had not, and concluded that paranoia was really a rare form of schizophrenia.

In the United Kingdom, the term 'paranoia', in its technical sense, had almost fallen into disuse by mid-century. Mayer-Gross, Slater and Roth, in the second edition of *Clinical Psychiatry* (1960), wrote off the condition as of 'merely historic interest'. These authors' views proved influential and in the United States in 1977 we find Gregory and Smeltzer echoing them. Later, in the United Kingdom, the *British Medical Journal* (1980) said that 'paranoia is no longer a fashionable term'. Yet the third edition of *Clinical Psychiatry* (Slater and Roth, 1969) had taken a very different line and endorsed the concept of paranoia with its encapsulated delusions and also of paraphrenia.

In *The International Statistical Classification of Diseases*, eighth edition (ICD8, 1968), paranoia was an *extremely* rare condition, while in ICD9 it had become simply rare. In the meantime, in DSMI (1952) paranoia was described in traditional terms and 'paranoid state' approximated to paraphrenia. In DSMII paranoid disorders (except paranoid schizophrenia) were grouped as 'paranoid states' (a loose amalgam of paranoia and paraphrenia) but it was questioned whether they were distinct from schizophrenia. DSMIII added confusion by describing paranoid disorders as characterized only by persistent delusions of persecution or delusional jealousy while still providing a rather half-hearted description of Kraepelinian paranoia. It also presented an unconvincing subgroup of illnesses named 'shared paranoid disorder' (an attempt to describe *folie à deux*), 'acute paranoid disorder' (see Chapter 11) and 'atypical paranoid disorder'.

Lewis (1970) wrote a seemingly authoritative article on paranoia and paranoid which nevertheless tails off in inconclusiveness. Similar perplexity is displayed in another standard British work, Henderson and Gillespie's *A Textbook of Psychiatry for Students and Practitioners*, whose sixth edition (1944) endorses the paranoid psychotic disorders as entities and even includes paranoid schizophrenia with them. Yet by its ninth edition (Henderson and Batchelor, 1962) it rejects the 'cumbersome' Kraepelinian nosological grouping of paranoia, paraphrenia and paranoid schizophrenia.

Prior to DSMIII, Winokur (1977) had re-described paranoia under the name 'delusional disorder', basing his findings on a strict nosological approach of Kraepelinian type and the observation of case types. In 1980, Kendler somewhat elaborated Winokur's criteria and suggested a division into simple delusional disorder (without hallucinations) and hallucinatory delusional disorder – a distinction currently regarded as redundant. Soon after, the present author (Munro, 1982a) separately evolved a description of paranoia remarkably like that of Kraepelin and the above two authors, based on a study of a series of patients with monodelusional hypochondriasis (see Chapter 2). Like Winokur's, this contribution emphasized subtypes of paranoia based on specific delusional contents.

Thus, by 1982, Winokur, Kendler and this writer had separately concluded that, despite all the intervening confusion since Kraepelin's death, paranoia existed, was much less rare than had been believed, and was readily diagnosable on empirically derived criteria. In addition, the present author presented evidence for treatability (see Chapter 13).

DSMIIIR agreed and its description of 'delusional (paranoid) disorder' was largely that of Kraepelinian paranoia except that 'nonprominent' hallucinations were allowed. The illness is distinct from affective and schizophrenic disorders. ICD10 (1992–93) has a very similar description and DSMIV differs only slightly from DSMIIIR.

So, despite its vicissitudes, paranoia, delusional (paranoid) disorder or simply delusional disorder, is now officially recognized and is increasingly being diagnosed. A more optimistic approach to treatment is giving an added incentive to seek out and carefully diagnose cases.

The clinical subtypes of paranoia

While paranoia was struggling to re-establish its credentials, its subtypes, especially erotomania and pathological jealousy, were enjoying a somewhat spurious independent existence, and these two entities will now be considered briefly.

Erotomania. As Enoch and Trethowan (1979) have shown, cases of apparent erotomania have been described since classical times. Kraepelin (1921) revived attention to it by designating erotomania as a subtype of paranoia. His typical patient was a middle-aged female disappointed in love, a description similar to that of Bianchi (1906). Kretschmer (1927) developed this stereotype of old maids developing a psychosis due to unrequited love and Hart (1921) actually referred to 'old maid's insanity'.

The psychiatrist most identified with the description of erotomania was de Clérambault, whose work was published posthumously in 1942. Despite his own insistence to the contrary, his 'pure' variety of erotomania is now regarded as synonymous with the Kraepelinian subtype of paranoia as accepted by DSMIV and ICD10. De Clérambault's secondary type of erotomania is best regarded as a complicating feature of another disorder such as schizophrenia (Segal, 1989).

In recent years, it has been demonstrated that erotomanic delusions can occur in men (Taylor, Mahendra and Gunn, 1983), who are more likely to act out their delusions (Goldstein, 1987). Also, cases of homosexual erotomania have been reported (Dunlop, 1988; Signer, 1989).

Pathological jealousy. Jealousy is as old as mankind but as Mullen (1991) points out, what was, in Western society at least, a socially acceptable reaction to infidelity has, at least in a proportion of cases, come to be regarded as evidence of psychopathology. While there has, for a very long time, been an appreciation of the difference between 'normal' or 'understandable' jealousy and the pathological variety, much of the literature on the subject is unclear as to the nature of that pathology.

Kraepelin (1899) clearly described cases of paranoid/delusional disorder in which jealousy was the predominant theme and he noted that this picture could arise in individuals addicted to drugs such as cocaine, as well as in alcoholics. An association between alcohol abuse and morbid jealousy was described as early as 1847 by Marcel and has been recorded by others, for example Langfeldt (1961) and Shepherd (1961) who also found an association with cocaine and amphetamine addictions.

Brierly (1932) and East (1936) confirmed the long-held impression of the dangerousness of pathological jealousy by showing that up to a quarter of *sane* murderers killed out of jealousy; and Mowat (1966), studying murderers who had been found criminally insane, estimated that 12 per cent of the males and 15 per cent of the females were motivated by jealousy. Indeed, the forensic aspects of morbid jealousy are a highly important aspect of the subject.

Freud (1958a) theorised that unconscious homosexual feelings were the basis for delusions of jealousy but subsequent workers, for example Langfeldt (1961), Shepherd (1961) and Vauhkonen (1968), found no support for this in their studies, although the last-named did report that a considerable number of his patients had other types of sexual dysfunction.

Retterstøl (1967) has provided one of the very few follow-up studies of pathological jealousy, involving 18 patients with 'jealousy-paranoiac psychosis', who were interviewed from $2\frac{1}{2}$ to 18 years after the initial diagnosis was made. His results suggest a more benign course than is usually reported: 11 out of 18 patients were delusion-free at review, but since the majority were classed as 'reactive psychosis, paranoiac', one has to speculate whether they would now be regarded as true delusional disorder cases.

In 1987, DSMIIIR included a monodelusional jealousy presentation as one of the subtypes of paranoia. Now, as 'delusional disorder, jealous subtype', this concept is enshrined in DSMIV and ICD10. The term 'Othello syndrome' (Schmeideberg, 1953; Enoch and Trethowan, 1979), often used as a synonym for pathological, especially delusional, jealousy, is confusing and should be avoided in clinical descriptions.

Paraphrenia

This disorder remained in ICD9, where it was said to be a 'paranoid psychosis in which there are conspicuous hallucinations, often in several modalities. Affective symptoms and disordered thinking, if present, do not dominate the clinical picture and the personality is well preserved.' (The category also subsumed involutional paranoid state and late paraphrenia.) This indicated that some psychiatrists in Europe and the United Kingdom still used the diagnosis, but it is rarely mentioned nowadays in the United States. It was not included in DSMIII, DSMIIIR or DSMIV, and in fact its last official recognition in the USA was in the 1945 *Statistical Manual for the Use of Hospitals for Mental Diseases* (American Psychiatric Association), tenth edition. Now, it has also disappeared from ICD10.

In 1960, Jackson commented that the diagnosis of paraphrenia was still commonly used in Britain and, in 1988, Black, Yates and Andreasen (1988) made the same comment, although they may have been referring specifically to 'late' paraphrenia. Yet, in 1970, Lewis said that paraphrenia was an uncommon diagnosis in Britain.

Much of the literature on paraphrenia is as contradictory as this indicates and it would be easy to conclude (if we did not have the example of paranoia to compare with) that paraphrenia must be something of a chimera to cause such uncertainty. Yet, as a practising clinician, this writer sees cases which closely agree with Kraepelin's description of paraphrenia and there are not a few fellow psychiatrists who feel the same way. Until ICD9 there was at least an official recognition of this viewpoint and Kendler and Tsuang (1981) stated, 'The followup results in general support Kraepelin's division of the paranoid psychotic disorders into three groups . . . Of these paranoid psychotic patients with bizarre delusions and/or hallucinations, about half go on to develop symptoms of thought disorder and personality deterioration (i.e. Kraepelin's paranoid dementia praecox) and half never develop such symptoms (i.e. Kraepelin's paraphrenia).'

If experts in the field believe the condition exists, why is it so widely ignored? There is no doubt that Kraepelin himself found paraphrenia more difficult to defend than paranoia and even before his death, Mayer (1921) had published a follow-up study of 78 cases of paraphrenia diagnosed in Kraepelin's own clinic. More than half the cases had deteriorated to other psychiatric diagnoses, but 28 of them had remained apparently paraphrenic. Subsequent writers have tended to stress the deteriorated cases and since then paraphrenia has often been regarded as a stage on the way to schizophrenia. A serious problem is that there has been no extensive case-series study on paraphrenia (except for 'late' paraphrenia – see Chapter 8) in the past half century.

The jury may still be out in the case of paraphrenia, but in the present era when diagnostic issues are much more alive than for a very long time, there is no question that its validity will be tested in many more scientific ways than ever before. There are those of us who believe that its existence will be vindicated just as paranoia's was. To this end. the writer and two of his colleagues, A. Ravindran and L. Yatham (personal communication, 1997), have undertaken a case-finding study which, in our view, vindicates our opinion that paraphrenia is a separate and recognisable disorder (see Chapter 7).

Late paraphrenia

In the sixth edition of his textbook (1899), Kraepelin introduced another delusional psychosis – presenile delusional insanity – which (despite the 'presenile') did not occur until the age of 55 or over and was not related to an organic aetiology. Bleuler (1950) later grouped these with schizophrenia (as he also grouped paraphrenia).

In the United States, presenile delusional insanity was accepted as an official diagnosis by the American Psychiatric Association until the emergence of DSMI in 1952, when it was combined with involutional melancholia to form 'involutional psychotic reaction' (presumably a mixture of severe affective and paranoid/delusional cases). In DSMII (1968), 'involutional paranoid state' was a return to the more Kraepelinian description of presenile delusional insanity and emphasized lack of marked schizophrenic thought disorder.

DSMIII refers to involutional melancholia and involutional paranoid disorder in its index, but they are not described in the text so are presumably regarded as *passé*. 'Atypical paranoid disorder' covers any case not described in the rest of its (unsatisfactory) paranoid disorder section. DSMIIIR's index mentions involutional melancholia but not involutional paranoid disorder, but there was a category of psychotic disorder not otherwise specified (NOS) which could, for some clinicians, allow some consideration of delusional disorders in the elderly.

ICD8 had a category of 'involutional paranoid state' but this is also called 'involutional paraphrenia' and is described as a paranoid variety of involutional psychotic reaction, without the conspicuous thought disorders typical of schizophrenia. ICD9 had paraphrenia, which also included 'involutional paranoid state'/'late paraphrenia'. ICD10 has 'other persistent delusional disorders', a residual category which can be used for all chronic delusional disorders not meeting the criteria for paranoid/ delusional disorder, which could include paraphrenia.

In the meantime, in England in the 1950s, Roth and his colleagues (Roth, 1955) had introduced the concept of 'late paraphrenia', an illness beginning in the sixties, seventies or even later and characterized by highly systematized delusions, while hallucinations in clear consciousness were also common.

This diagnosis continues to be used widely in Britain (and may be why Black, Yates and Andreasen (1988) thought that paraphrenia was a common term there), but argument about its separate diagnostic status continues. Post (1966) and Holden (1987) argue against it, Grahame (1984) argues for it but says there is a considerable overlap with schizophrenia, and Soni and colleagues (1988) see similarities with schizophrenia but argue for its separateness. Late paraphrenia is discussed further in Chapter 8.

Schizophrenia and paraphrenia are, in this author's belief, separate disorders, but in advanced old age their presentations become so similar that it is probably no longer worthwhile arguing for a diagnostic differentiation on noninvestigative clinical findings alone. This aspect is considered elsewhere (see Chapter 9).

Late onset schizophrenia

As noted, Kraepelin did not exclude late onset cases of schizophrenia from his category of dementia praecox, but after his time many psychiatrists were unwilling to label a case schizophrenic if a psychotic illness began after the age of 45. This has led to tortuous attempts to diagnose late onset functional psychoses without actually calling them schizophrenic.

Nowadays, there is an increasing acceptance of late onset schizophrenia but it is still not altogether clearly defined. Most authorities agree that it is more likely to be paranoid schizophrenia with bizarre delusions and hallucinations but relatively little disturbance of thought form. It is much more common in females, and a family history of schizophrenia is often absent. Response to neuroleptic medication is frequently good.

It will save a great deal of semantic manoeuvring if this category becomes widely accepted and, if it is, it could be that, as suggested previously, no real differentiation can be made between first onset schizophrenia and paraphrenia in the very elderly, except possibly by neuroinvestigative means.

Delusional misidentification syndromes – background aspects

While the conditions discussed until now have been regarded at various times as belonging to a group of paranoid or delusional disorders, it is now time to introduce a relative stranger which presently has no categorical status.

In 1923, Capgras and Reboul-Lachaux presented the case of a middle-aged woman who believed that her close relatives had been replaced by identical doubles as part of a plot to steal her property. Their description has become the prototype for the concept of the delusional misidentification syndromes, of which a number of varieties has been enumerated (Christodoulou, 1978). These will be considered later in Chapter 9.

As time has gone on, purely psychological theories of aetiology have gradually given way to increasing evidence of organic brain factors in aetiology (Cummings, 1985), including organically determined problems in facial recognition (Ellis and Young, 1990), although Fleminger (1992) adduces evidence for a combination of psychological and organic brain factors as causation.

Some authors, for example de Pauw, Szulecka and Poltock (1987), have noted parallels between the delusional misidentification syndromes and paranoid/delusional disorder, and this is discussed further in Chapter 10. Interestingly, in the more recent literature there have been a small number of reports of successful treatment of Capgras or Frégoli phenomena with pimozide (de Pauw, Szulecka and Poltock, 1987; Passer and Warnock, 1991; Tueth and Cheong, 1992), which provides further tentative evidence for features in common (see Chapter 13). Later, it will be argued that the group of delusional misidentification syndromes warrants a niche in the official diagnostic category of delusional disorders.

Reactive and periodic psychoses

Alongside the discussions and arguments about schizophrenia and para-noid/delusional disorders there is a parallel controversy as to whether there is yet another mixed group of psychotic disorders, characterized on the one hand by periodicity and on the other by brief duration and the presence of precipitating stress factors. As will be seen in Chapter 11, there is a good deal of uncertainty and authors often use the concepts of periodicity and reactiveness synonymously, which is not always appropriate. It is necessary to provide a very brief background to these two types of disorder so that subsequent discussion of their characteristics may be more intelligible.

Periodic psychoses

Cycloid psychosis is the archetype of the periodic psychosis. Leonhard (1961) has provided the most comprehensive description of the illness and proposes three subtypes (which are mentioned in Chapter 11). Fish (1974) took a more simplistic approach and described cycloid psychosis as an illness with schizophrenic symptoms and a manic–depressive course. Some episodes may be precipitated by stressors but most seem to arise sponta-neously (Cutting, 1990). Most authors agree that the prognosis for an individual episode is usually good.

Some authors (e.g. Cutting, 1990) have proposed that cycloid psychosis is an atypical form of bipolar disorder, while others (e.g. Perris, 1988; Fish, 1974) see it as a separate disorder. What is important in our context is that an episode of cycloid psychosis may be very difficult to separate from schizophrenia (Leonhard, 1961; Fish, 1974), schizoaffective disorder (Per-ris, 1988) or paranoid disorder (Crammer, 1959). At present, cycloid psychosis is not included in DSMIV or ICD10 and therefore, as Perris (1988) points out, is often misdiagnosed as schizophrenia or schizoaffec-tive disorder for want of awareness of its existence.

Reactive psychoses

Here we have a category of illness in which an episode of psychosis is precipitated by stress and then tends to clear up once the stress is removed. The acute picture is often mistaken for schizophrenia or for delusional disorder (DSMIII had a separate category of acute paranoid disorder) but rapid resolution of symptoms usually makes the differentiation clear. DSMIV (1994) describes 'brief psychotic disorder' and ICD10 (1992–93) has 'acute and transient psychotic disorders', both of which essentially capture the essence of the brief reactive psychosis but, as will be discussed in Chapter 11, show evidence of misunderstandings in both cases.

The ancestors of the reactive psychoses are, on the one hand, 'hysterical psychosis' (Hirsch and Hollander, 1969; Cavenar, Sullivan and Maltbie, 1979) and, on the other, *'bouffée délirante'* (Pichot, 1986), but the picture has been complicated by the addition of the Scandinavian concept of reactive or 'psychogenic' psychosis, an illness described (Retterstøl, 1978) as occurring in constitutionally predisposed personalities as the result of stress and tending to clear up over time (in some cases as much as two years). Unfortunately there is controversy about the latter (Dahl, 1987) and a substantial proportion of cases has been shown to deteriorate to schizophrenia or bipolar disorder (Jauch and Carpenter, 1988). The implications of some of these controversial concepts are further discussed in Chapter 11.

Paranoid personality disorder

Many German psychiatrists regard the presence of a foregoing personality disorder, especially of the paranoid or 'sensitive' type, to be a frequent antecedent of paranoid/delusional disorder, thereby making the latter more 'understandable'. There seems little doubt that many patients with established paranoid/delusional disorder did have odd or eccentric premorbid personalities, but this has never been shown to 'explain' the psychotic illness.

DSMIV (1994) and ICD10 (1992–93) take an atheoretical approach and describe this personality disorder in terms of identifiable features rather than postulated causation and mental mechanisms. It is included in the 'cluster A' personality disorders (along with schizoid and schizotypal personality disorders), recognising that it is often difficult to diagnose a specific personality disorder when it is more a question of recognising in a given individual a predominance of particular traits which are shared in differing proportion by several personality disorders.

If delusions appear, the diagnosis is then superseded by that of a psychotic disorder. Certain authors (e.g. Kretschmer, 1927; Akhtar, 1990) suggest that paranoid personality disorder is genetically and phenomenologically related to the paranoid/delusional disorders. There is little scientific evidence for this, although the impression is a persistent one. A study by Kendler and Gruenberg (1982) is the nearest approach to an empirical confirmation, although it seems to show a link between paranoid personality disorder and 'schizophrenia and related disorders', rather than just paranoid/delusional disorders alone.

Conclusions regarding the delusional disorders

To sum up and, in the process, to oversimplify, the following are suggested as relevant to the illnesses which have been discussed:

(1) Paranoia/delusional disorder is a disorder in its own right whose description is still, to some extent, clouded by archaic concepts. It is considerably more common than usually thought.

(2) Paraphrenia is well delineated in the older literature and, if given a modern description (see Chapter 7), is probably as distinguishable from schizophrenia as is delusional disorder.

(3) Paranoid schizophrenia is a well-established diagnosis but, instead of retaining it as a subtype of schizophrenia, serious consideration should be given to returning it to the category of delusional disorders, as Kraepelin originally proposed.

(4) Late paraphrenia may well be a continuation into old age of paraphrenia.

(5) Late onset schizophrenia is simply schizophrenia beginning in an older individual. The more advanced the age, the more difficult it is to differentiate late paraphrenia from it, and at that age this clinical differentiation may no longer be useful.

(6) Cycloid and reactive psychoses should be distinguished clearly from each other (see Chapter 11) and should never be confused with delusional disorder.

(7) Delusional misidentification syndromes are currently an orphan group of disorders which, in this author's view, should be included among the delusional disorders. At this time they are of great interest because they show considerable promise of providing significant neuropathological evidence about the genesis of certain delusions.

(8) Paranoid personality disorder, despite its name, has no place among the paranoid/delusional disorders, although some cases (along with other group A personality disorders) may develop psychotic symptoms under certain conditions, at which point the disorder may enter into the paranoid spectrum (see Chapter 7).

Despite the apparent 'separateness' of the above diagnoses, a recurring theme in the literature is that a proportion of cases from virtually any of them may change rapidly or gradually to schizophrenia. We must therefore be aware that these disorders can either be illnesses in their own right or, less commonly, may be a temporary stage in a deteriorative pathological process.

Notes on phenomena associated with delusions

Introduction

Delusional disorder is so called because a delusional system is the most prominent feature of its symptomatology. Of course, delusions are not the only feature of the illness, and delusional disorder is only one of many psychiatric conditions associated with delusions. However, a relatively unique feature of this particular condition is that, because of the encapsulated nature of the false beliefs, delusional and nondelusional aspects of mental function appear to coexist in the same individual, thereby giving a golden opportunity to compare and contrast them. Sadly, until now, little or no systematic research has been carried out on this or other aspects of delusions in delusional disorders.

Delusions are regarded as one of the most characteristic elements of all the psychotic illnesses and in both the *Diagnostic and Statistical Manual of Mental Disorders*, fourth edition (DSMIV) and the *International Statistical Classification of Diseases*, tenth edition (ICD10) they are among the symptoms cited as most essential to the diagnosis of schizophrenia and delusional disorder.

It is a widely held view that delusions are qualitatively different from normal ideas or beliefs and have an all-or-nothing quality. The DSMIV definition appears to confirm this viewpoint. It states that a delusion is

A false belief based on an incorrect inference about external reality that is firmly sustained despite what almost everyone else believes and despite what constitutes incontrovertible and obvious proof or evidence to the contrary. The belief is not one ordinarily accepted by other members of the person's culture or subculture (e.g. it is not an article of religious faith). When a false belief involves a value judgment, it is regarded as a delusion only when the judgment is so extreme as to defy credibility. Delusional conviction occurs on a continuum and can sometimes be inferred from an individual's behaviour.

The definition goes on to say that 'It is often difficult to distinguish between a delusion and an overvalued idea (in which case the individual has an unreasonable belief or idea but does not hold it as firmly as is the case with a delusion).' This now seems to imply a somewhat less than black-and-white view of delusion. Also, the phrase 'delusional conviction occurs on a continuum' suggests that there is no clear division between delusional and nondelusional thinking.

This inconsistency of definition is not unique to DSMIV but pervades the whole topic, and the clinician has to use what knowledge is at hand, but should be aware that even 'official' descriptions, as in DSMIV and ICD10, are very unsatisfactory. Experts in the field frequently express their frustration by making comments like: 'Delusions remain enigmatic even after many years of research' (Butler and Braff, 1991) and 'A review such as this is limited by the heterogeneity of the data surveyed. Studies span several decades and have widely differing methodologies' (Flint, 1991). As yet, we even continue to have problems at times in distinguishing between delusions and overvalued ideas (McKenna, 1984).

This task has become increasingly difficult as traditional systems of nosology and diagnostics have been challenged and subsequently altered, and it is unfortunately true that the working clinician still does not have a more reliable yardstick than the DSM/ICD definitions of delusion (Sedler, 1995).

A very great problem in interpreting the findings of studies on delusions in psychiatric illness is that diagnostic criteria for cases under investigation are frequently imprecise or outdated and diagnostic categories are mixed. As has been remarked for delusional disorder, systematic studies are few, case series are always brief and the quality of the diagnosis is very often in doubt, especially in reports prepared prior to the late 1980s. There have been a number of excellent reviews on delusions in recent years, including Arthur (1964), Winters and Neale (1983), Butler and Braff (1991), Maher (1992), and Garety and Hemsley (1994), but despite their perceptive approach and the distinguished work done by many of these authors, the conclusions still usually contain a caveat similar to that of Butler and Braff (1991): 'A reliable and valid method of quantifying and characterizing delusions is needed so that the impact of changes in diagnostic nomenclature can be empirically validated.'

Phenomenology and psychopathology of delusions

Phenomenology in the field of medicine at large is the study of phenomena pertaining to health and disease. A prime aim of that study is to allow us to cluster such phenomena into characteristic and recurring patterns to provide us with a description of syndromes or illnesses. When these descriptions appear to have both validity and reliability, we can then utilize the methods of pathological investigation to enquire into causation, to establish prognosis and, by extension, to determine the effectiveness of a specific treatment on a discrete illness. This approach has been the mainstay of scientific progress in the field of physical disease since the mid-nineteenth century, and nowadays is subserved by many sophisticated investigative disciplines representing a wide biological spectrum.

Phenomenology and pathology in the physical domain aim to be empirical and atheoretical. However, like any branch of science they are open to speculation, hypothesis and argument and, also like science in general, their data will change as new facts become available. The living brain has been so inaccessible until recently and our methods for studying it have been so crude and at such a distance from the actual pathology, that we have had to rely on conjecture which all too often becomes dogma.

Many modern psychiatrists loosely think of phenomenology in the field of psychiatry as being directly analogous to phenomenology elsewhere in medicine, but this is rarely the case. One can make direct measurements of temperature or blood pressure, study the constituents of blood or urine, interpret the appearances of a radiograph or examine a tissue sample under the electron microscope. One cannot make observations like this on thought disorder, hallucinations or delusions: we cannot even, at this stage, agree with any degree of exactness just what these epiphenomena are.

A traditional approach in the phenomenological study of the psychiatric patient has therefore been to use *empathy* (Gruhle, 1915; Jaspers, 1963) as a way in which to understand how a patient thinks or feels at a given time and how, for example, a delusional idea may affect him or her. This does not mean that we actually understand the delusion or the illness to which it belongs: instead, we have 'felt' ourselves into the patient's mind and can recognize something different from our own 'normal' experience, and can therefore appreciate both this abnormal phenomenon and the individual's response to it.

There is no question that this method has enabled us, over many years, to build up a useable descriptive phenomenology in psychiatry but it is easy to see how subjective the approach is, how open it may be to the observer's bias and theoretical approach, and how difficult it will be for different observers to agree on what they have observed and what to call it. And this is exactly what has happened, with different schools of psychiatry using their own exclusive jargons and deriving their own particular inferences.

When DSMIII appeared in 1980, it avowed to be as dogma-free as possible and it and its successors have been at pains to adopt a rather bleakly reductionistic approach to the description of psychiatric phenomena and psychiatric illness. This seems to have coincided with a growing trend in many centres outside as well as inside the USA, and ICD10 has largely followed the DSM lead. The result, for many psychiatric phenomenologists, is an abrupt split in ideology between the discipline's past and its present. This has *not* occurred in the classificatory aspect of psychiatric illnesses, especially for the major psychiatric disorders, since it has gone back largely to Kraepelinian principles.

In psychiatry, our traditional concepts of delusion largely stem from the work of Karl Jaspers (1883–1969), whose writings have been enormously influential in the areas of phenomenology and psychopathology (Jaspers, 1963).

Jaspers' definition of delusion consisted of the following criteria:

(1) That the belief is held with extraordinary conviction and with profound subjective certainty.
(2) That it is maintained against the effect of other experiences and of convincing counter-argument.
(3) That it is impossible with regards to its content.

He insisted that delusions were incapable of being modified, and proposed that the incorrigibility of the delusional belief was the individual's outstanding protection against internal mental collapse (i.e. the pit prop, despite being bent and cracked, might still prevent the mine roof from falling). The primary delusion, in Jaspers' view, was caused by a hypothetical disease process in the brain: it was therefore not susceptible to *psychological* enquiry. The characteristics of the premorbid personality might provide the material for the delusional content, but again could not explain the delusion itself.

These views remain extremely influential in psychiatry and still form the basis of teaching about delusions in many textbooks. A more recent author (Mullen, 1979) adopts a similar definition and is widely cited in the modern psychiatric literature when delusions are described. He characterized delusions as follows:

(1) They are held with absolute conviction.
(2) The individual experiences the delusional belief as self-evident and regards it as of great personal significance.
(3) The delusion cannot be changed by an appeal to reason or by contrary experience.

(4) The content of delusions is unlikely and often fantastic.
(5) The false belief is not shared by others from a similar socio-economic group.

This is very similar to the definitions subsequently adopted by DSMIV (1994) and ICD10 (1992–93), both of which emphasize the profound dichotomy between delusion and normal belief. But, as will be seen a little later, recent investigations challenge all of the criteria mentioned above.

Jaspers described several types of delusions and although these descriptions are used much less nowadays, they are briefly presented here so that the reader who is not familiar with them will have some experience with the terms if he or she comes across them in reading. Also, we tend to throw such terms around quite carelessly in discussion and it is as well to have an accurate grasp of their original intentions (Sims, 1988). Jaspers divided delusions into *primary* and *secondary* forms. The *primary delusion* is seen by Jaspers as arising from an abnormality of brain and is not understandable (by the standards of current knowledge). Primary delusions were further divided into four types, thus:

(1) Autochthonous delusion (or 'delusional intuition'), which is phenomenologically similar to the sudden appearance of a normal idea, especially an inspirational idea. The idea appears fully-formed ('autochthonous' means 'sprung from the soil') with strong intuitive certainty. This process occurs in a single step.
(2) Delusional percept is a normal perception imbued with delusional meaning. Although the belief is false, it has tremendous significance for the individual, and the perception remains unaltered even though it now has a profound new interpretation for the patient. A distinction is made here from the 'delusional misinterpretation', which is an adaptation of a percept to fit in with other delusional beliefs. The process of developing a delusional percept is said to occur in two stages, the first in which a belief is perceived as especially meaningful and the second in which it becomes invested with delusional significance.
(3) Delusional atmosphere (also known as delusional mood or Wahnstimmung) is the phenomenon where the person senses the world to be subtly changed in a significant way. This may be allied with 'delusional awareness' in which there is a heightened appreciation of atmosphere. There is a feeling of anticipation often associated with perplexity and apprehension and this, not uncommonly, is relieved when the delusion crystallizes out.

(4) Delusional memory (or 'retrospective delusion'): this resembles an autochthonous delusion or a delusional percept but it presents as a false memory. The individual claims to remember something which did not happen and will attest to this with conviction. Oddly, this (apparently the least of Jaspers' four types of primary delusion) has become rather important as a concept of late. Current controversies about 'recovered memories' and the 'false memory syndrome' have raised a spectre for mental health professionals and for patients' relatives of being unjustly accused of sexual and other misdemeanours long after the acts have allegedly been done. Most such cases are not related to delusions or to delusional disorders, but when an accusatory paranoid individual makes persistent and fanatically pursued charges, it might be very difficult in some cases for the accused person to prove his or her innocence.

Secondary delusion is said to be understandable in the patient's present mood or circumstances, in relation to peer group beliefs or as a long-term outgrowth of personality factors or cumulative life experiences. It is suggested as being an unconscious manoeuvre on the part of the patient to 'explain' his or her other symptoms and thereby to gain psychological relief. While this may be the commonsense explanation, in practice it is often difficult to separate primary and secondary delusions and, at most, the delusional content may appear to be explained, but not the delusional mechanism.

In academic and clinical discussion, the primary–secondary distinction often comes to the fore but it has largely been abandoned in recent clinical classificatory systems, especially DSMIV and ICD10.

Delusions and nosology

Attempts have been made to classify psychotic disorders according to the content of their delusions (Sinha and Chaturvedi, 1989). This has only limited usefulness (Maher, 1992). There is, for example, some evidence that delusions in schizophrenia may have certain distinguishing qualities (Schneider, 1959) and, of course, once the diagnosis of delusional disorder has been made, the specific delusional theme can then usefully distinguish the different subtypes (e.g. jealousy, erotomania, somatic, etc.) (Munro, 1995). Also, in major depression with delusions, the mood-congruent quality of the delusions, with themes of poverty, self-deprecation and nihilism, may be very characteristic (Cutting, 1985). But, in general, one gets only limited help in diagnosing illness by relying solely upon the delusional content: it is rare to be able to identify the illness unmistakably by this alone.

Recent experimental work on delusions

Recent work on delusions is cautionary, since many of our dearly held beliefs do not hold up to detailed examination. For example, it now appears that:

(1) Delusions are not rigidly fixed but can fluctuate in intensity over time, even in the absence of treatment (Alloy, 1988).

(2) Delusional incorrigibility does not appear to be absolute (Garety and Hemsley, 1994) and evidence is growing that, under certain circumstances, delusional thinking can be modified (e.g. by cognitive therapy) (Kingdon, Turkington and John, 1994). Also, it has come to be realised that maintaining a strong belief against opposing evidence is not by itself abnormal but is instead a common normal human trait (Ross and Anderson, 1982).

(3) Some clinicians continue to maintain that delusions are relatively impervious to medications but there is little *bona fide* research in this area and common sense observation seems to indicate that, with an increasing repertoire of new treatments this is less and less so. That is not to say that we necessarily *cure* delusions, but certainly effective treatment in major mood disorder or delusional disorder can allay them to the point where they are either no longer evident or interfere minimally with normal functioning.

(4) Delusions are not, as we often believe, absolute yes/no entities. Instead there is growing evidence that they are complex, multidimensional phenomena (Kendler, Glazer and Morgenstern, 1983). To some extent these dimensional elements are independent of each other and can either co-vary or vary independently.

(5) A delusion is not necessarily a blind belief and some delusional individuals can think about them and even collaborate with investigators in measuring them (David, 1990).

(6) Bizarreness of a delusion is rapidly losing its credibility as a distinguishing feature (Flaum, Arndt and Andreasen, 1991; Mojtabai and Nicholson, 1995). In delusional disorder, where the delusions are usually tightly structured and defended with, at times, exquisite pseudo-logic, the premise may still be quite bizarre despite what

DSMIV and ICD10 say. (For example, one of the author's patients who was unhappy with the outcome of a cosmetic operation on his nose was convinced that his future well-being depended on his having a second operation to shorten his neck.)

Any clinician working with delusional patients must be aware of the many challenges to his or her traditional understanding and definition of delusion. It is not the purpose of this book to discuss the complex experimental and theoretical situation which exists in relation to delusions but we should be aware of the uncertainty of our understanding of delusions and the implications this may have in our diagnosis of the disorders with which they are associated. In the meantime, until more scientifically validated and clinically applicable definitions appear, we are mostly left with the clearly unsatisfactory descriptions of delusions in DSMIV and ICD10.

No widespread agreement about the origin of delusions exists and many theoretical positions are under exploration (Maher, 1988; Harper, 1992; Garety and Hemsley, 1994). Interestingly, while so much uncertainty remains, a slowly increasing and clinically relevant literature on the behavioural–cognitive treatment of delusions is emerging (Kingdon, Turkington and John, 1994; Fowler and Morley, 1989). And, from the psychiatrist's viewpoint, an exciting recent development is the collaboration between psychologists, psychiatrists and brain scientists in studying the delusional misidentification syndromes (see Chapter 9), where findings particularly pertinent to clinical practice are beginning to emerge.

Some idea of the complex interweaving of historical and current concepts of delusions can be obtained from a number of excellent recent publications (Garety and Hemsley, 1994; Manschrek, 1995; Roberts, 1992; Schifferdecker and Peters, 1995; Spitzer, 1990, 1992). The psychoanalytic approach has been advanced lately by writers such as Aronson (1989) and Freeman (1990) but the influence of this school on the medical approach to patients with delusions is very small at the present time.

Sociodemographic theories of the origin of delusions were once influential, but recent evidence has suggested that societal influences are mainly on the content of delusions rather than on their form, and cannot explain their aetiology. Studies on the phenomena of koro (Ang and Weller, 1984), amok (Gelder and colleagues, 1996) and delusional hypochondriasis (Munro, 1982b) appear to demonstrate this. Considerations of delusions as atavistic phenomena and as misapplications of normal mental mechanisms in unfamiliar modern situations (Schlager, 1995) are beguiling, but as yet almost entirely hypothetical.

At this time we are beginning to see very early indications of possible effects of brain pathology on psychopathology, including the generation of delusions (Cummings, 1985; McAllister, 1992) and this is an area of exciting new potential because of the variety of new investigative tools becoming available.

Delusions in clinical practice: a practical approach

When reading the literature on delusions, one is aware that a great deal of it was written before any of the therapeutic advances in psychiatry that began in the mid-1950s. These advances have revolutionised our approach to psychiatric illness and to the patient, have introduced the necessity for scientific methodology in the study and treatment of such illness, and incidentally have taken away the leisure to study cases *in extenso*.

It is only in the past generation that real experimentation has begun in the field of phenomenology, including the study of delusions. In psychiatric texts, there are still confident descriptions of what delusions are, the phenomena related to them, and how they appear. Unfortunately the confidence is not always allied to consistency, so that definitions, nomenclature and descriptions overlap, vary subtly and become embroiled in the philosophies to which their protagonists adhere, even when they claim to be eclectic. Much of this, as already noted, has still not been applied to psychiatric practice.

In the clinical world, where there is now an imperative to treat as efficiently and effectively as possible, we must have a practical working approach which allows us to recognize a delusion, place it in a diagnostic context, and treat it along with the other phenomena that make up the particular illness in an individual patient. Sims (1988) makes an interesting and rather bold observation when he says, 'there is usually very little difficulty for the observer in deciding whether a false belief is a misinterpretation of the facts based on false reasoning, or a delusion'. That statement is difficult to prove and, at the very least, requires the word 'skilled' to be interpolated before the word 'observer'. However, it does seem to be true that the experienced and insightful clinician develops some sense of when a belief is likely to be false and is held with delusional intensity, and this has to be the starting point of the clinical observation that the patient is deluded.

Of course, the patient does not make this observation, because his belief to him is a self-evident truth. What is it then that alerts the psychiatrist to the likelihood that he is dealing with a delusion and therefore a delusional illness? It is rarely one factor, but rather an accumulation of nuances which leads him to these conclusions. The following are suggested as indicators, no one of which is pathognomonic, but an accumulation of which is increasingly suggestive.

(1) The patient expresses an idea or belief with unusual persistence or force.
(2) That idea appears to exert an undue influence on his or her life, and the way of life is often altered to an inexplicable extent.
(3) Despite his profound conviction, there is often a quality of secretiveness or suspicion when the patient is questioned about it.
(4) The individual tends to be humourless and oversensitive, especially about the belief.
(5) There is a quality of *centrality*: no matter how unlikely it is that these strange things are happening to him, the patient accepts them relatively unquestioningly.
(6) An attempt to contradict the belief is likely to arouse an inappropriately strong emotional reaction, often with irritability and hostility.
(7) The belief is, at the least, unlikely.
(8) The patient is emotionally overinvested in the idea and it overwhelms other elements of his psyche.
(9) The delusion, if acted out, often leads to behaviours which are abnormal and/or out of character, although perhaps understandable in the light of the delusional beliefs.
(10) Individuals who know the patient will observe that his belief and behaviour are uncharacteristic and alien. (The exception is when a *folie à deux* is occurring – see Chapter 10.)
(11) There may be associated features such as suspicion, hauteur, grandiosity, evasiveness, threatening behaviour or eccentricity, as well as hallucinations, thought disorder, mood change, etc. Acting out of the delusion (Buchanan, 1993) and violent behaviours associated with delusions (de Pauw and Szulecka, 1988) may also occur.
(12) Perhaps most important, the delusion will occur in the setting of a psychiatric disorder whose other features are characteristic: the delusion and its content will be strongly coloured by the specific nature of that disorder. Also, the delusion will usually respond to the treatment appropriate to the disorder.

When the clinician has observed an accumulation of several of the above elements in a particular patient, he or she must be highly suspicious that delusions are present.

Conclusions

We may be thankful that DSMIV and ICD10 both recognize delusional disorder, since that illness (in its previous incarnation as paranoia) was in almost total eclipse until its reacceptance in 1987 by DSMIII. Nevertheless, the official diagnostic systems remain niggardly in restricting the category to only one illness. In Part II we shall look at paranoia/delusional disorder in detail, but then in Part III a case will be made for a 'paranoid spectrum' which includes several illnesses in addition to delusional disorder.

The history of paranoia, and especially of its exclusion from the standard diagnostic canons of the mid-twentieth century, makes salutary reading. Careless diagnostic practice allowed it to be overshadowed by other illnesses, especially schizophrenia. Despite recent advances in our recognition of psychiatric disorders, similar things still happen today. Paraphrenia, once equally accepted as a separate diagnosis alongside paranoia, is still under the shadow of schizophrenia. Delusional misidentification syndrome (DMS), which has many similarities to delusional disorder, is simply in limbo, with no classificatory recognition whatsoever.

Adequate definition of illness is essential before worthwhile research can be carried out on it, and lack of good clinical research ultimately means poor patient care. There also needs to be much more applied research in the field of delusions and related phenomena so that we can become more skilled at recognising the phenomena, and eliciting the psychopathology of the paranoid spectrum disorders.

The rest of this book will attempt to define the features and the boundaries of these illnesses and will differentiate them from other conditions with superficial similarities which do not form part of the same group.

References

Akhtar, S. (1990). Paranoid personality disorder: a synthesis of developmental, dynamic and descriptive features. *Am. J. Psychother.* **44**: 5–25.

Alloy, L.B. (1988). Expectations and situational information as co-contributors to covariation assessment: a reply to Goddard and Allen. *Psychol. Rev.* **95**: 299–301.

Ang, P.C. and Weller, M.P.I. (1984). Koro and psychosis. *Br. J. Psychiat.* **145**: 335.

Aronson, T.A. (1989). Paranoia and narcissism in psychoanalytic therapy. *Psychoanalyt. Rev.* **76**: 329–351.

Arthur, A.Z. (1964). Theories and explanations of delusions: a review. *Am. J. Psychiat.* **121**: 105–115.

Berner, P. (1965). *Das Paranoische Syndrom.* Berlin: Springer.

Bianchi, L. (1906). *A Textbook of Psychiatry.* Transl. J. H. Macdonald. London: Baillière, Tindall & Cox.

Black, D.W., Yates, W.R. and Andreasen, N.C. (1988). Delusional (paranoid) disorders. *In Textbook of Psychiatry*, ed. J. A. Talbot. pp. 391–396. Washington, DC: American Psychiatric Press Inc.

Bleuler, E. (1950). *Dementia Praecox or the Group of Schizophrenias.* Transl. J. Ainkia. New York: International Universities Press.

Brierly, H.C. (1932). *Homicide in the United States.* New York: Chapel Hill.

British Medical Journal (1980). Leading article: paranoia and immigrants. **281**: 1513–1514.

Buchanan, A. (1993). Acting on delusion: a review. *Psychol. Med.* **23**: 123–134.

Butler, R.W. and Braff, D.L. (1991). Delusions: a review and integration. *Schizophr. Bull.* **17**: 633–647.

Capgras, J. and Reboul-Lachaux, J. 1923 L'illusion des 'sosies' dans un délire systématisé chronique. *Bull. Soc. Clin Méd. Mentale* **2**: 6–16.

Cavenar, J.O., Sullivan, J.L. and Maltbie, A.A. (1979). A clinical note on hysterical psychosis. *Am. J. Psychiat.* **136**: 830–832.

Christodoulou, G.W. (1978). Syndrome of subjective doubles. *Am. J. Psychiat.* **135**: 249–251.

De Clérambault, G. (1942). *Les Psychoses Passionelles. Oeuvre Psychiatrique.* Paris: Presses Universitaires.

Crammer, J.L. (1959). Periodic psychoses. *Br. Med. J.* **1**: 545–549.

Cummings, J.L. (1985). Organic delusions: phenomenology,anatomical correlations and review. *Br. J. Psychiat.* **146**: 184–197.

Cutting, J. (1985). *The Psychology of Schizophrenia.* Edinburgh: Churchill Livingstone.

Cutting, J. (1990). Relationship between cycloid psychosis and typical affective psychosis. *Psychopathology* **23**: 212–219.

Dahl, A.A. (1987). Problems concerning the concept of reactive psychoses. *Psychopathology* **20**: 79–86.

David, A.S. (1990). Insight and psychosis. *Br. J. Psychiat.* **156**: 798–808.

Diagnostic and Statistical Manual of Mental Disorders, 1st edn. (DSMI) (1952). Washington, DC: American Psychiatric Association.

Diagnostic and Statistical Manual of Mental Disorders, 2nd edn. (DSMII) (1968). Washington, DC: American Psychiatric Association.

Diagnostic and Statistical Manual of Mental Disorders, 3rd edn. (DSMIII) (1980). Washington, DC: American Psychiatric Association.

Diagnostic and Statistical Manual of Mental Disorders, 3rd edn. revised (DSMIIIR) (1987).Washington, DC: American Psychiatric Association.

Diagnostic and Statistical Manual of Mental Disorders, 4th edn. (DSMIV) (1994). Washington, DC: American Psychiatric Association.

Dunlop, J.L. (1988). Does erotomania exist between women? *Br. J. Psychiat.* **153**: 830–833.

East, W.N. (1936). *Medical Aspects of Crime.* London: Churchill.

Ellis, H.D. and Young, A.W. (1990). Accounting for delusional misidentifications. *Br. J. Psychiat.* **157**: 239–248.

Enoch, M.D. and Trethowan, W.H. (1979). *Uncommon Psychiatric Syndromes.* Bristol: John Wright and Sons.

Fish, F.J. (1974). *Clinical Psychopathology.* ed. M. Hamilton. Bristol: John Wright and Sons.

38   *Outline and introduction*

Flaum, M. Arndt, S. and Andreasen, N.C. (1991). The reliability of 'bizarre' delusions. *Compr. Psychiat* **32**: 59–65.

Fleminger, S. (1992). Seeing is believing: the role of 'preconscious' perceptual processing in delusional misidentification. *Br. J. Psychiat.* **160**: 293–303.

Flint, A.J. (1991). Delusions in dementia: a review. *Neuropsychiat. Clin. Neurosci.* **3**: 121–130.

Fowler, D. and Morley, S. (1989). The cognitive-behavioural treatment of hallucinations and delusions: a preliminary study. *Behav. Psychother.* **17**: 267–282.

Freeman, T. (1990). Psychoanalytical aspects of morbid jealousy in women. *Br. J. Psychiat.* **156**: 68–72.

Freud, S. (1958a). *Extracts from the Fleiss Papers*, standard edn., vol. 1, pp. 173–280. London: Hogarth Press.

Freud, S. (1958b). *The Case of Schreber*, complete works, vol. 12, ed. J. Strachey. London: Hogarth Press.

Garety, P.A. and Hemsley, D.R. (1994). *Delusions: Investigations into the Psychology of Delusional Reasoning*. Maudsley Monograph No. 36. Oxford: Oxford University Press.

Gelder, M., Gath, D., Mayou, R. and Cowen, P. (1996). *Oxford Textbook of Psychiatry*, 3rd edn., p. 191. Oxford: Oxford University Press.

Goldstein, R.L. (1987). More forensic romances: de Clérambault's syndrome in men. *Bull. Am. Acad. Psychiat. Law* **15**: 267–274.

Grahame, P.S. (1984). Schizophrenia in old age (late paraphrenia). *Br. J. Psychiat.* **145**: 493–495.

Gregory, I. and Smeltzer, D.J. (1977). *Psychiatry*. Boston: Little, Brown.

Gruhle, H.W. (1915). Self-description and empathy. *Ztsch. ges. Neurol. Psychiat* **28**: 148–155.

Harper, D.J. (1992). Defining delusion and the serving of professional interests: the case of 'paranoia'. *Br. J. Med. Psychol.* **65**: 357–369.

Hart, B. (1921). *The Psychology of Insanity*. Cambridge: Cambridge University Press.

Henderson, D.K. and Batchelor, I.R. (1962). *Henderson and Gillespie's Textbook of Psychiatry*, 9th edn. London: Oxford University Press.

Henderson, D.K. and Gillespie, R.D. (1944). *A Textbook of Psychiatry for Students and Practitioners*, 6th edn. London:Oxford University Press.

Hirsch, S.J. and Hollander, M.H. (1969). Hysterical psychosis: clarification of the concept. *Am. J. Psychiat.* **125**: 81–87.

Holden, N.L. (1987). Late paraphrenia or the paraphrenias? A descriptive study with a 10–year follow-up. *Br. J. Psychiat.* **150**: 635–639.

Huber, G. (1992). The phenomenological approach to major psychoses in Europe during the past several decades. *Neurology, Psychiatry, Brain Res.* **1**: 49–53.

International Statistical Classification of Diseases, 8th edn. (ICD8) (1968). Geneva: World HealthOrganization.

International Statistical Classification of Diseases, 9th edn. (ICD9) (1978). Geneva: World HealthOrganization.

International Statistical Classification of Diseases, 10th edn. (ICD10) (1992–3). Geneva: WorldHealth Organization.

Jackson, D.D. (1960). *The Etiology of Schizophrenia*. New York: Basic Books.

Jaspers, K. (1963). *General Psychopathology* (originally published 1913), transl. J. Hoenig and M. Hamilton. Manchester: University of Manchester Press.

Jauch, D.A. and Carpenter, W.T. (1988) Reactive psychosis I. Does the pre-DSMIII concept define a third psychosis? *J. Nerv. Ment. Dis.* **176**: 72–81.

Kahlbaum, K. (1863). *Die Gruppirung der psychischen Krankheiten.* Danzig: Kafemann.

Kendler, K.S. (1980). The nosologic validity of paranoia (simple delusional disorder). *Arch. Gen. Psychiat.* **37**: 699–706.

Kendler, K.S., Glazer, W.M. and Morgenstern, H. (1983). Dimensions of delusional experience. *Am. J. Psychiat.* **140**: 466–469.

Kendler, K.S. and Gruenberg, A.M. (1982). Genetic relationship between paranoid personality disorder and the 'schizophrenic spectrum' disorders. *Am. J. Psychiat.* **139**: 1185–1187.

Kendler, K.S. and Tsuang, M.T. (1981). Nosology of paranoid schizophrenia and other paranoid psychoses. *Schizophrenia Bull.* **7**: 594–610.

Kingdon, D., Turkington, D. and John, C. (1994). Cognitive behaviour therapy of schizophrenia. *Br. J. Psychiat.* **164**: 581–587.

Kolle, K. (1931). *Die Primäre Verrücktheit.* Leipzig: Thieme.

Kraepelin, E. (1896). *Lehrbuch der Psychiatrie,* 5th edn. Leipzig: Barth.

Kraepelin, E. (1899). *Lehrbuch der Psychiatrie,* 6th edn. Leipzig: Barth.

Kraepelin, E. (1903–04). *Lehrbuch der Psychiatrie,* 7th edn. Leipzig: Barth.

Kraepelin, E. (1909–13). *Lehrbuch der Psychiatrie,* 8th edn. Leipzig: Barth.

Kraepelin, E. (1921). *Manic-Depressive Insanity and Paranoia.* Transl. R. M. Barclay, (1976). New York: Arno Press.

Kretschmer, E. (1927). *Der sensitive Beziehungswahn,* 2nd edn. Berlin: Springer.

Langfeldt, G. (1961). The erotic jealousy syndrome. A clinical study. *Acta Psychiat. Scand.* Suppl. 151.

Leonhard, K. (1961). Cycloid psychoses – endogenous psychoses which are neither schizophrenia nor manic-depressive. *J. Ment. Sci.* **107**: 633–648.

Lewis, A. (1970). Paranoia and paranoid: a historical perspective. *Psychol. Med.* **1**: 2–12.

Maher, B.A. (1988). Anomalous experience and delusional thinking: the logic of explanations. In *Delusional Beliefs,* ed T.F. Oltmanns and B.A. Maher, pp. 15–33 New York: John Wiley.

Maher, B.A. (1992) Delusions: contemporary etiological hypotheses. *Psychiat. Ann.* **22**: 260–268.

Manschrek, T.C. (1995). Pathogenesis of delusions. *Psychiat. Clin. N. Am.* **18**: 213–229.

Marcel, C.N.S. (1847). De la folie causée par l'abus des boissons alcooliques. Paris: Thesis p. 461.

Mayer, W. (1921). Über paraphrene Psychosen. *Z. Ges. Neurol. Psychiat.* **71**: 187–206.

Mayer-Gross, W., Slater, E. and Roth, M. (1960). *Clinical Psychiatry,* 2nd edn., pp. 264–265. London: Cassell & Co.

McAllister, T.W. (1992). Neuropsychiatric aspects of delusions. *Psychiat. Ann.* **22**: 269–277.

McKenna, P.J. (1984). Disorders with overvalued ideas. *Br. J. Psychiat.* **145**: 579–585.

Mojtabai, R. and Nicholson, R.A. (1995). Interrater reliability of ratings of delusions and bizarre delusions. *Am. J. Psychiat.* **152**: 1804–1806.

Mowat, R.R. (1966). *Morbid Jealousy and Murder.* London: Tavistock Publications.

Mullen, P. (1979). Phenomenology of disordered mental function. In *Essentials of Post-graduate Psychiatry*, ed. P. Hill, R. Murray and G. Thorley, pp. 25–54. London: Academic Press.

Mullen, P.E. (1991). Jealousy: the pathology of passion. *Br. J. Psychiat.* **158**: 593–601.

Munro, A. (1982a). Paranoia revisited. *Br. J. Psychiat.* **141**: 344–349.

Munro, A. (1982b). *Delusional Hypochondriasis.* Clarke Institute of Psychiatry Monograph No. 5. Toronto: Clarke Institute of Psychiatry.

Munro, A. (1995). The classification of delusional disorders. *Psychiat. Clin. N. Am.* **18**: 199–212.

Munro, A. and Mok, H. (1995). An overview of treatment in paranoia/delusional disorder. *Can. J. Psychiat.* **40**: 616–622.

Passer. K.M. and Warnock, J.K. (1991) Pimozide in the treatment of Capgras' syndrome: a case report. *Psychosomatics* **32**: 446–448.

de Pauw, K.W. and Szulecka, T.K. (1988). Dangerous delusions.Violence and the misidentification syndromes. *Br. J. Psychiat.* **152**: 91–96.

de Pauw, K.W., Szulecka, T.K. and Poltock, T.L. (1987). Single case study. Frégoli syndrome after cerebral infarction. *J. Nerv. Ment. Dis.* **175**: 1–6.

Perris, C. (1988). The concept of cycloid psychotic disorder. *Psychiat. Developm.* **1**: 37–56.

Pichot, P. (1986). The concept of 'bouffée délirante' with special reference to the Scandinavian concept of reactive psychosis. *Psychopathology* **19**: 35–43.

Post, F. (1966). *Persistent Persecutory States of the Elderly.* Oxford: Pergamon Press.

Retterstøl, N. (1966). *Paranoid and Paranoiac Psychoses.* Springfield IL: Thomas.

Retterstøl, N. (1967). Jealousy–paranoiac psychoses: a personal follow-up study. *Acta Psychiat. Scand.* **43**: 75–107.

Retterstøl, N. (1978). The Scandinavian concept of reactive psychosis, schizophreniform psychosis and schizophrenia. *Psychiatr. Clin.* **11**: 180–187.

Roberts, G. (1992). The origins of delusion. *Br. J. Psychiat.* **161**: 298–308.

Ross, L. and Anderson, C.A. (1982). Shortcomings in the attribution process: on the origins and maintenance of erroneous social assessment. In *Judgment Under Uncertainty: Heuristics and Biases*, ed. K. Kahneman, P, Slovic and A. Tversky, pp. 129–152. New York: Cambridge University Press.

Roth, M. (1955). The natural history of mental disorder in old age. *J. Ment. Sci.* **101**: 281–301.

Schifferdecker, M. and Peters, U.H. (1995). The origin of the concept of paranoia. *Psychiat. Clin. N. Am.* **18**: 231–249.

Schlager, D. (1995). Evolutionary perspectives on paranoid disorder. *Psychiat. Clin. N. Am.* **18**: 263–279.

Schmeideberg, M. (1953) Some aspects of jealousy and of feeling hurt. *Psychoanal. Rev.* **40**: 1–16.

Schneider, K. (1959). *Clinical Psychopathology*, pp. 161–162. New York: Grune and Stratton.

Sedler, M.J. (1995). Understanding delusions. *Psychiat. Clin. N. Am.* **18**: 251–262.

Segal, J.H. (1989). Erotomania revisited: from Kraepelin to DSMIIIR. *Am. J. Psychiat.* **146**: 1261–1266.

Shepherd, M. (1961). Morbid jealousy: clinical and social aspects of a psychiatric symptom. *J. Ment. Sci.* **107**: 687–753.

Signer, S.F. (1989). Homo-erotomania. *Br. J. Psychiat.* **154**: 729 (letter).

Sims, A. (1988). *Symptoms in the Mind: An Introduction to Descriptive Psychopathology*, p.82. London: Baillière Tindall.

Sinha, V.K. and Chaturvedi, S.K. (1989). Persistence of delusional content among psychotics over consecutive episodes. *Psychopathology* 22: 208–212.

Slater, E. and Roth, M. (1969). *Clinical Psychiatry*, 3rd edn, pp. 294–295. London: Baillière, Tindall & Cassell.

Soni, S.D., Mallik, A., Mbatia, J. and Shrimankar, J. (1988). Late paraphrenia. *Br. J. Psychiat* 153: 719–720 (letter).

Spitzer, M. (1990). On defining delusions. *Comp. Psychiat.* 31: 377–397.

Spitzer, M. (1992). The phenomenology of delusions. *Psychiat. Ann.* 22: 252–259.

Statistical Manual for the Use of Hospitals for Mental Diseases, 10th edn. (1945). Utica: Utica StateHospitals Press.

Stengel, E. (1957). Concepts of schizophrenia. *Br. Med. J.* 1: 1174–1176.

Taylor, P., Mahendra, B. and Gunn, J. (1983). Erotomania in males. *Psychol. Med.* 13: 645–650.

Tueth, M.J. and Cheong, J.A. (1992). Successful treatment with pimozide of Capgras syndrome in an elderly male. *J. Geriat. Psychiat. Neurol.* 5: 217–219.

Vauhkonen, K. (1968). On the pathogenesis of morbid jealousy. *Acta Psychiat. Scand.* Suppl. 202.

Winokur, G. (1977). Delusional disorder (paranoia). *Comp. Psychiat.* 18: 511–521.

Winters, K.C. and Neale, J.M. (1983). Delusions and delusional thinking in psychotics: a review of the literature. *Clin. Psychol. Rev.* 3: 227–253.

Part II

Descriptive and clinical aspects of paranoia/delusional disorder

The paranoid disorders may be the third great group of functional psychoses, along with affective disorder and schizophrenia.
Dr Kenneth S. Kendler
(Archives of General Psychiatry, 1982, 39:890–902)

'Lumping and splitting' is a process that goes on all the time in science, as categories are grouped and regrouped, divided and dispersed. In medicine, diagnoses are changing constantly as new evidence accrues and old knowledge proves inadequate. At the same time the diagnoses are being included with, or separated from, other diagnoses according to their apparent similarities and contrasts. All of this is an attempt to provide a taxonomy of illness, a coherent schema so that illnesses can be classified with some degree of coherence. It is an ever-evolving dynamic process, since new information is continually revealing fresh relationships or exploring false similarities.

In 1900, paranoia was a well-accepted diagnosis. By 1950 it was vanishing from the psychiatric textbooks. In the year 2000 it will again be a widely recognized illness. How can this be? Much of the answer is to do with inappropriate lumping and especially to do with the over-enthusiastic and slipshod diagnosis of schizophrenia in the mid-twentieth century, particularly in the United States. Although it is very different from schizophrenia, superficial similarities led paranoia to be included under that rubric for many years. Research on, and knowledge of, paranoia almost totally dried up during that time.

Since the 1980s the picture has changed dramatically. Paranoia – now delusional disorder – is enjoying an increasingly lusty independent existence, but this gives rise to a strange situation. Much of our knowledge, and a great deal of our theorising on the topic, comes from almost a century back and new information which is beginning to appear is difficult to square with the old. The literature, to say the least, is confusing. The present book is an attempt to draw together the past and the present and to make a coherent picture of delusional disorder for the clinician and the researcher.

But not only was delusional disorder unfortunately lumped with schizophrenia; it itself turns out to be a 'lump' – a disorder with several different subtypes. There was good awareness of this 100 years ago, but as the central concept was forgotten the individual varieties developed lives of their own and their relationship to the centre was forgotten. So, the present author's work must show first the independence of delusional disorder as a diagnosis, and secondly that it is an accumulation of subtypes whose similarities are greater than their differences.

This section therefore gives an overall presentation of delusional disorder with a description of its most important background features and then looks in some detail at the subtypes, especially those with somatic, jealousy, erotomanic, persecutory, and grandiose delusional contents. There is repeated emphasis on the fact that the diagnosis of delusional disorder is made on certain characteristic features, including the *form* of the delusional system. The *content* of the delusion is used mainly to describe which subtype a particular individual's illness belongs to.

2

Paranoia or delusional disorder

Introduction

By the end of the nineteenth century, paranoia was well established as a psychiatric illness and was regarded as being not uncommon. Yet, as has been described in Chapter 1, it all but vanished as a diagnosis during the middle of the twentieth century. That process, and the subsequent rehabilitation of the concept, has already been discussed in some detail.

Renamed 'delusional disorder', paranoia was firmly reinstated in 1987 by DSMIIIR and it is fully accepted under this title in DSMIV (1994) and ICD10 (1992–93). It is increasingly being diagnosed, but because of its long absence from the canon, it is not necessarily familiar to all psychiatrists.

What is meant by paranoia?

This chapter will describe an illness characterized by a stable and persistent delusional system which is relatively encapsulated and which, in many cases, leaves much of the personality surprisingly intact, allowing a considerable degree of social functioning to persist. The individual clings to the delusion with fanatical intensity and nearly always spurns any suggestion that he or she is ill. Hallucinations may occur but are usually less prominent than in schizophrenia: when they are present their themes tend to be congruent with the delusional belief. The illness is chronic, often in fact lifelong, but it does not have the principal characteristics of schizophrenia as stipulated by criterion A for schizophrenia in DSMIV.

Paranoia was renamed 'delusional disorder' in DSMIIIR because of the considerable confusion of terminology in English-speaking psychiatry. For example, 'paranoia' denotes the specific psychiatric syndrome which will shortly be described, but is often confused with the term 'paranoid' which, according to usage can mean a group of psychotic illnesses, a particular personality disorder or, nowadays, most often a layman's description of angry, suspicious attitudes.

Some years ago, Fish (1974) pointed out that most English-speaking psychiatrists used 'paranoid' synonymously with 'persecutory' and Case No. 1 (below) has been selected as typical of what many people, lay and professional, would consider to be paranoia. The patient who is described here does indeed suffer from paranoia/delusional disorder and the main delusion has a persecutory content, but contents of a nonpersecutory nature are at least as common in other cases of the disorder. Fish contended that 'paranoid' should have the general implication of 'delusional' but common parlance insists that 'paranoia' and 'paranoid' usually mean suspicion with irritability and there need be no suggestion of delusional thinking. Nowadays, the only official 'paranoid' diagnosis in DSMIV and ICD10 is paranoid personality disorder which, by definition, is prohibited from being associated with delusions. So, DSMIIIR, and now DSMIV and ICD10, have abandoned the term paranoia and refer to the illness as delusional disorder. In this chapter, paranoia and delusional disorder are employed interchangeably, but the latter is now the more usual term.

Let us illustrate some of the features of paranoia/delusional disorder with an actual case. As has been said, this individual typifies many of the features which the lay person identifies with 'paranoia'.

Case No. 1   Delusional disorder, persecutory subtype

A 38-year-old man was arrested by the police after he had held up a local radio station for several hours, threatening staff members with a loaded pistol and demanding that a message written by him be transmitted to the public. After a tense standoff situation, the police finally persuaded him to lay down his gun and he was taken into custody. Early in the ensuing legal process he was found unfit to plead because of mental disorder and he has remained in a locked forensic psychiatric facility since.

About four years before the hold-up incident he had moved to another city. While there he had contact with a prostitute and, several months later, he suddenly developed the conviction that she had transmitted a fatal disease to him. He never decided what this disease was, but he went to several medical clinics where he was thoroughly tested and no evidence of physical illness was ever found. This did not allay his belief and, in fact, his delusional system gradually elaborated, so that he now believed that he had been deliberately infected as part of a world-wide plot which involved Jewish people. He thought that the plot was designed to infect the whole population and cause widespread death. He ruminated end-lessly about this, could not work, was constantly agitated and in fear, and became increasingly angry that no one would listen to him or believe him. He eventually returned home and brooded for many months before deciding to storm the radio station, his rationale being that he must warn the general population before he died.

The patient is a man of average intelligence who comes from a troubled family with a considerable history of violence. In his earlier years he abused a number of drugs, especially LSD and marijuana, and he had been in trouble with the police several times for carrying weapons. Despite this, for several years prior to the onset of his symptoms he appeared to have settled down and was gainfully employed, but he led a quite solitary existence.

During his current prolonged stay in a forensic unit he has totally maintained his delusional beliefs and has consistently refused treat-ment. In many ways he is a model patient, and he takes an acute interest in his own case. He has instigated three unsuccessful pleas against incarceration and has conducted himself reasonably in court, except that he has consistently maintained that he is the victim of a plot and that he will, if necessary, use violence to expose it. Despite continuing good physical health he cannot be convinced that he is not dying of his imagined disease. There was a one month period when he was legally required to take neuroleptic medication and temporarily he appeared less concerned about his delusions and even admitted he felt better. Then the requirement to take treatment was cancelled and he immediately refused to take any more, al-though his distressing symptoms rapidly returned to their former level.

Having introduced delusional disorder with a case description, let us now look at the official symptom description as portrayed in DSMIV and, almost identically, in ICD10.

In DSMIV (1994), the primary symptom is non-bizarre delusion(s) of at least one month's duration. (The definition of 'non-bizarre' is becoming increasingly difficult to sustain and is currently falling out of favour – see Chapter 1.) Criterion A, which emphasizes the deteriorative features of schizophrenia, has not been met and, apart from the direct effects of the delusion(s), functioning is relatively unimpaired and behaviour (at least in public) is not notably odd. Any associated mood disturbances are fleeting and the illness is not due to the direct effects of a substance of abuse or a medication.

Several subtypes are described, according to the predominant delusional theme. These are: erotomanic; grandiose; jealous; persecutory; somatic; and mixed and unspecified.

ICD10 describes the main feature as a delusion or set of related delusions not typical of schizophrenia and the general criteria for schizophrenia are absent. In this case, the delusions are supposed to be present for at least three months. Persistent hallucinations are not present but occasional transitory hallucinations of non-Schneiderian type may occur. Mood symptoms may be present but, when absent, the delusions still persist. The illness is not secondary to an organic mental disorder or to psychoactive substance abuse.

The same subtypes are described according to delusional content, but additional terms are supplied in ICD10, such as litigious, self-referential and hypochondriacal.

Overall features of delusional disorder (Munro, 1995)

In general terms, we can think of delusional disorder as having the following features:

(1) It is a primary disorder, not secondary to another psychiatric condition (however, see p.61).
(2) It is a stable disorder characterized by the presence of delusions to which the patient clings with extraordinary tenacity.
(3) The illness is chronic and frequently lifelong.
(4) The delusions are logically constructed and internally consistent.
(5) The disorder is a monomania, with a predominant, persistent theme.
(6) Despite the monodelusional aspect, the content of the delusion varies from patient to patient, although a limited number of themes predominate.
(7) The delusions do not interfere with general logical reasoning

(although within the delusional system the logic is perverted) and there is usually no general disturbance of behaviour. If disturbed behaviour does occur it is directly related to the delusional beliefs.

(8) Many cases appear to arise in the setting of a markedly abnormal personality.

(9) Hallucinations may or may not be present (there has been some dispute about this but, as noted, DSMIV and ICD10 allow non-prominent hallucinations).

(10) The individual experiences a heightened sense of self- reference. Events which, to others, are nonsignificant are of enormous significance to him or her and the atmosphere surrounding the delusions is highly charged.

Despite the encapsulation of the delusional system and the relative sparing of the personality, the patient's way of life is likely to become more and more overwhelmed by the dominating effect of the abnormal beliefs. Since the hallucinations are usually not very intrusive they may be difficult to distinguish from delusional misinterpretations or illusions. Contrary to what DSMIV and ICD10 say, other hallucinations of an olfactory or coenaesthepathic nature can occur in addition to auditory phenomena.

The illness seems to affect males and females approximately equally, although data are sparse, and the age of onset can be from adolescence to extreme old age. There is some evidence that males may be at risk of earlier initiation, and that in advanced old age female cases predominate. Many patients are unmarried, separated, divorced or widowed and the premorbid personality is said to be isolative and asocial. Even so, the condition is sometimes – perhaps often – compatible with marriage and continued employment, although many of these individuals are noted to be eccentric or fanatical.

Deafness is conventionally regarded as an aetiological factor in 'paranoid' disorders, and this seems to be documented to some extent for late paraphrenia (Kay and Roth, 1961) and for paranoid schizophrenia (Cooper, Curry and Kay, 1974) but less well for delusional disorder. Thomas (1981), on the other hand, found little increase in paranoid symptoms generally with deafness and Watt (1985) noted no association between deafness and paranoid states of middle life. Gloag (1980) has reminded us that deafness of varying degrees is so common in middle and older age that associations with mental illness can only be made by comparison with a suitable control group, something that is rarely done. With regard to blindness there is even less evidence but Guensberger,

Fleischer and Sipkovska (1977) say that paranoid psychoses are much rarer in the blind than in the deaf.

Although it may fluctuate in intensity from time to time, delusional disorder is a very chronic condition and appears permanent in many cases. In some patients it is possible that a long and insidious onset may result in the mimicking of a cluster A personality disorder (e.g. paranoid, schizoid or schizotypal personality disorder), but significant premorbid personality abnormalities do seem common (Kendler, Masterson and Ungaro, 1984). Men especially are liable to have a previous history of psychoactive substance abuse or head injury, suggesting the possibility of a subtle underlying organic brain abnormality in these patients (Munro, 1982).

Onset may be gradual or acute. In either instance, the patient may identify, sometimes vehemently, a precipitating factor which is difficult to confirm or deny. (For example, patients with infestation delusions who respond well to treatment may continue to insist that they actually did have a real infestation at the outset.) Some individuals successfully keep their delusions hidden or even utilize them: for example, grandiose apocalyptic beliefs may fit very well with the views of certain extreme religious sects, and one suspects that a small minority of the most persistent and intrusive 'community activists' are driven by delusional fervour. Other people become prominent by acting out their delusions, sometimes colliding with the authorities as a result. Erotomanic 'stalking' of women is an increasingly publicised example of such antisocial behaviour (Zona, Sharma and Lane, 1993).

One of the most unique and striking features of delusional disorder is the way in which the patient can move between delusional and normal modes of thought and behaviour (Munro, 1992). In the former, the individual is overalerted, preoccupied with the delusional ideas, and gives a sense of being remorselessly driven. In contrast, the normal mode is associated with relatively calm mood, reasonable range of affect, neutral conversation with an ability to be engaged in everyday topics, and some capacity for pursuit of normal activities. But the delusional beliefs are always nearby, ready to pounce and to change the person's whole attitude and demeanour. A comparison with Dr Jekyll and Mr Hyde is not totally inappropriate.

In the delusional mode, thought form is relatively normal but the abnormal thought content predominates and is associated with profound illogicality. However, the individual may be capable of marked focusing of attention and, since he is constantly rehearsing his delusional beliefs, is often able to present them forcefully and convincingly. There is no effective insight and because a delusion is held with extraordinary conviction, any attempt at contradiction is met with anger and disdain, the latter reflecting some degree of grandiosity in many cases.

Delusional contents

Subtypes of delusional disorder are based on the particular delusional content and when a diagnosis of delusional disorder has been made, one proceeds to assign the subcategory according to the DSMIV and ICD10 descriptions.

Within the subcategories, further subsets can occur. For instance, the somatic (hypochondriacal) subtype includes delusions of skin infestation, convictions of bodily abnormalities or of emitting a foul odour: in the persecutory subtype a proportion of the individuals becomes increasingly litigious. These various manifestations will each be dealt with separately.

Other delusional contents may occur but appear to be relatively rare and it is interesting that the repertoire of delusional beliefs in delusional disorder is fairly limited. Although the concept of 'nonbizarre' delusions has already been criticised (Flaum, Arndt and Andreasen, 1991; Mojtabai and Nicholson, 1995), it seems possible that the delusional disorder patient may be able to reject those beliefs which are truly improbable, since he retains some degree of insight within the more normal aspects of the personality.

There is more contact with reality than in most other psychotic conditions because the patient is only partially 'insane'. It is almost pathognomonic of the disorder that the individual refuses to see a psychiatrist. This seems to be partly the result of his unstinting belief in his delusions which to him are totally factual and therefore do not need any meddling from an interfering specialist. He will more than readily visit a cosmetic surgeon if he thinks his physical appearance is abnormal (Hawes and Bible, 1990) or a lawyer if he thinks his colleagues are persecuting him (Rowlands, 1988), but great pressure usually has to be put on him before a psychiatric consultation can take place. Apart from the delusional rejection of any psychiatric aetiology, however, there also seems to be in many cases some degree of nondelusional awareness that exposure to a psychiatrist may pose a threat to his belief system. This suggests some 'normal' insight but unfortunately it gets in the way of the patient's receiving appropriate help.

More so than with other psychiatric illnesses, the delusional content decides which type of agency the patient comes in contact with, either voluntarily or involuntarily. That, in turn, often dictates the context within which the psychiatrist, if involved, has to work. Naturally, there will be differences in the way in which cases will be handled: for example, one patient may have to be seen in a forensic psychiatric setting, having already passed through law enforcement and judicial processes, because he attacked his wife in a jealous frenzy, whereas another patient has been referred from a dermatological clinic to a psychiatric clinic in the same hospital for a diagnostic assessment. Whatever the administrative process, if a delusional disorder is diagnosed, then the illness *form* is relatively constant whatever the context, despite the profound differences in delusional *content* from patient to patient. The psychiatrist should be skilled at recognising the illness form despite the confounding variables because the treatment approach depends on that. Essentially the treatment is the same whatever the actual nature of the delusional belief.

Illnesses associated with delusions: the differential diagnosis of delusional disorder

Although paranoia is increasingly known as 'delusional disorder', the great majority of illnesses associated with delusions do not belong to this specific category. Regrettably, even this statement is somewhat controversial, as some authorities regard 'delusional disorders' as all psychiatric illnesses with delusions, subcategorising them according to the underlying syndrome, which might be schizophrenia, severe mood disorder, or even organic mental disorder (Berner, 1965; Retterstøl, 1966). On the other hand, DSMIV and ICD10 restrict the term 'delusional disorder' to paranoia, but unfortunately imply that this is the only illness within the category which, as will be argued elsewhere (see Chapters 7 and 9), is overly restrictive.

When considering a possible diagnosis of delusional disorder, the other principal illnesses with delusions which must be excluded are:

Paraphrenia
Paranoid schizophrenia
Other schizophrenias
Organic mental disorder, including mental disorders due to a
    medical condition
Psychoactive substance-induced organic mental disorders and
    withdrawal disorders
Psychotic disorders not elsewhere classified
Mood disorders with delusions
Delusional misidentification syndromes
Induced psychotic disorder or *folie à deux* (in which the beliefs
    are delusional although the patient is not truly deluded)

Several of the above are sufficiently important (and sometimes sufficiently ill-understood) to warrant separate consideration in the present volume and readers are advised to refer to the appropriate chapters dealing with them.

The following are mentioned only briefly here, since a detailed description is not warranted and can readily be obtained from the standard classificatory systems or textbooks.

Schizophrenias other than paranoid schizophrenia

In general, schizophrenia will present as a chronic psychotic illness marked by delusions and hallucinations, often widespread, fluctuating and with many themes. Mood disturbance and thought disorder are prominent, with flattened and/or inappropriate affect. Speech, reflecting thought disorder, is markedly disturbed, psychomotor behaviour is abnormal, and the individual's relationship to the world and to other people is severely distorted. Volition is affected, resulting either in impulsive or in negative behaviours. There is deterioration in lifestyle and in occupational functioning. Without treatment, many schizophrenics become chronic invalids. A family history of schizophrenia is often present. Occasionally, in the schizophreniform stage of schizophrenia, a picture like the well encapsulated delusional system of delusional disorder may occur but this usually disintegrates after a relatively short time.

Delirium

This is the result of a general medical illness and when full-blown is usually unmistakeable. When low grade or fluctuating there may be periods of near-full consciousness when delusions and hallucinations are present and a resemblance to delusional disorder or schizophrenia fleetingly occurs (Lipowski, 1980). Otherwise, the illness is characterized by reduced consciousness, cognitive and memory deficits and, at times, totally disorganised behaviour. These symptoms affect the patient, his thinking and his behaviour indiscriminately. The course is related to the underlying illness and the success of its treatment.

Dementia

There are many causes and presentations of dementia, but the two main clinical pictures are those of generalized, Alzheimer-type dementia and vascular (multi-infarct) dementia. The former usually has a gradual onset and the latter is often more sudden, with associated neurological abnor-malities. In the early stages of Alzheimer's disease, a picture apparently identical to delusional disorder may emerge before the dementing features are apparent, and the present author has seen a small number of cases of seemingly typical persecutory, erotomanic and somatic subtype delusional disorder which have, over a period of a year or two, developed increasing signs of dementia. One should therefore beware of the onset of an apparent functional psychosis of late life in an elderly individual, especially if the onset is relatively rapid and occurs in the setting of a previously well-balanced personality.

In the vascular type of dementia, depressive disorder is not uncommon and in severe cases may be associated with delusions which are often, not surprisingly, hypochondriacal but sometimes persecutory. One may also see frankly persecutory delusional states which may at times be linked to elements of misidentification (see Chapter 9). The presence of focal neur-ological signs is important in differential diagnosis but may not be clini-cally obvious in white matter lesions, which have assumed considerable importance in recent years.

Otherwise, dementia may be related to specific disorders such as head injury, HIV infection, Huntington's chorea, parkinsonism, Pick's disease, Creutzfeldt–Jakob disease, cerebrosyphilis and many others. Paranoid symptoms have been mentioned traditionally in Huntington's disease and grandiosity is commonly described in cerebrosyphilis and sometimes in Pick's disease, due to predominantly pre-frontal lobe involvement at cer-tain stages of these illnesses.

Note: individuals (especially male) who are significantly head injured at some stage in life but not severely demented seem to be excessively prone to develop delusional disorder years later.

Substance-induced psychotic disorder

This may occur in close time relationship to substance abuse or substance withdrawal and then clear up. In a proportion of cases following severe abuse there may be a persisting mental disorder occurring in clear con-sciousness and usually characterized by hallucinations, delusions or both. Thought disorder, if present, is not gross. Chronic dysphoria is not uncom-mon and a degree of avolition is quite frequently seen. Some deterioration of social and occupational activity occurs but is difficult to measure since the substance abuse itself usually adversely affects lifestyle. Irritability and ideas of reference may be present.

In some cases a frank and at times typical paranoia emerges and this may occur many years after the cessation of the substance abuse. The appearances may then be indistinguishable from delusional disorder, including the presence of typical subtype themes, unless other marked evidences of organic brain disorder are noted. When the latter are not present, a diagnosis of delusional disorder is probably justified, especially since such patients may respond to treatment like idiopathic cases.

Commentary on differential diagnosis

Schizophrenia and organically or substance-induced cerebral features should always be excluded as a routine in the differential diagnosis of delusional disorder but we have to accept that a patient with a history of substance abuse and/or head injury in the past may be excessively liable, possibly as a result of limited cerebral insults, to develop true delusional disorder at a later time.

Otherwise, none of the illnesses mentioned above has the tightly organised, chronic, monodelusional quality of paranoia/delusional disorder.

Non-delusional illnesses which may mimic delusional disorder: further differential diagnostic considerations

Having considered other illnesses characterized by delusions which have to be distinguished from paranoia, it is also important to mention certain non-delusional disorders which may bear a superficial resemblance to some of the subtypes of delusional disorder.

The most important of these is body dysmorphic disorder, an illness formerly known as dysmorphophobia, which is now an obsolete term. Body dysmorphic disorder, or BDD, is a chronic, nonpsychotic somatoform disorder in which there is a persistent, but nondelusional, subjective belief of bodily abnormality. The patient is convinced that the abnormality is obvious to others: in some cases a relatively minor physical abnormality does exist but this is totally insufficient to warrant the serious concern shown by the sufferers. The complaint is usually very specific and there is intense importuning for care from the specialists perceived by the patient as appropriate. This illness is considered in more detail in Chapter 12.

Other forms of somatoform disorder, notably somatization disorder and conversion disorder, may also superficially resemble delusional disorder, somatic subtype. A small number of apparent cases of eating disorder may actually be suffering from delusional disorder, but true eating disorder cases may present with beliefs about physical appearance that are so bizarre that it is easy to mistake them for delusions. Careful history-taking and differential diagnosis are essential here.

Equally, some cases of obsessive–compulsive disorder may have extremely persistent, quasi-delusional thoughts and fears regarding cleanliness, imagined physical illness, infidelity fears and so on. Usually, however, the patient has insight and resists the thoughts while, in contrast, delusional disorder patients are in total consonance with their beliefs (see Chapter 12).

From time to time there are reports of pathological jealousy of nonpsychotic type. The jealousy may be exceedingly severe and lead to profound limiting behaviour and even aggression towards the sexual partner. An obsessional element may again be important here (see Chapter 4).

Certain personality disorders can have features reminiscent of delusional disorder, especially the paranoid, schizoid and schizotypal varieties. In these, patients show features such as suspiciousness, ideas of reference, isolated and withdrawn behaviour, highly eccentric beliefs (for example about health and nontraditional treatments), marked interpersonal difficulties and difficulty with reality testing. Despite all of these, the patients are not psychotic and their ideas are not delusional (see Chapter 12).

It is extremely important to make careful diagnostic distinctions since it is rarely appropriate to prescribe neuroleptic drugs to any of the foregoing disorders. In fact, it has been the present author's unfortunate experience in the past to have to re-diagnose several cases labelled as 'paranoid' or 'delusional' illness who were actually suffering from obsessive–compulsive disorder. These individuals had been condemned for long periods to take neuroleptic medications which were totally inappropriate for them.

Finally, *folie à deux* must be mentioned (currently known as shared psychotic disorder in DSMIV and induced delusional disorder in ICD10) since it occurs in association with a significant number of cases of delusional disorder (9 out of 50 in the author's series). Again, the topic is considered in more detail later (see Chapter 10), but two aspects are underlined here. The first is the question of false corroborative evidence given by the *folie à deux* individual which may cause mistaken credence to be given to the deluded patient's complaints. The second relates to the specific treatment approach taken in cases of *folie à deux* (see p.189).

Considerations of aetiological factors in delusional disorder

Knowledge of aetiology in this condition is very limited and speculation ranges from the enthusiastic, viz. in psychoanalytic theory, to the near-nihilistic, as in Jaspers' 'ununderstandability' approach (Jaspers, 1963). Sadly, in the field of delusional disorders we still have great difficulty in delineating causative factors in a convincing fashion. This is in marked contrast to what is happening with the delusional misidentification disorders (see Chapter 9) which, in this author's view, are providing a model of what should be happening in the field of delusional disorder.

In this section a brief description of our scanty knowledge of aetiology will be set out in four areas: genetic speculations, organic factors said to be of importance, links with mood factors and finally, some further commentary on psychodynamic theories.

Genetic factors in delusional disorders

In a salutary article, Kendler (1987) clearly demonstrated the profound effects on calculations of family history patterns in psychiatric illness as the result of misdiagnosis among the probands. A relatively small proportion of misdiagnoses can lead to highly erroneous conclusions and nowhere is this truer than in delusional disorder. Prior to 1987, when paranoia was revived by DSMIIIR as delusional disorder, there was utter confusion about the definition and diagnosis of the illness, and very few older studies on its familial characteristics can now be read with any confidence. In fact, many can no longer be read with any real comprehension since definitions and classifications have changed so dramatically. In the past decade, the study of heredity in schizophrenia has been forging ahead though still hampered by difficulties in obtaining homogeneous samples. In the same period there has been little or nothing about the genetics of delusional disorder, and that may well be a consequence of the difficulties in gathering adequate series.

At the most basic level, that of actual genetic abnormalities, Axelson and Wahlström (1984) reported that approximately one-third of their patients with 'paranoid psychosis' had demonstrable chromosome aberrations as compared with a total lack of such abnormalities in their controls. Unfortunately, the nature of the diagnosis of paranoid psychosis is not clearly described and the meaning of the chromosomal findings is unexplained, so the finding remains an intriguing but opaque one.

Farmer, McGuffin and Gottesman (1987) studied DSMIII schizophrenia by a twin-concordance method and in the course of this found that both paranoid schizophrenia and paranoid disorders (especially paranoia) appeared less heritable than other forms of schizophrenia. They speculated that paranoid disorders might indeed be genetically separate: the difficulty here from our point of view is that these paranoid disorders are a mixed group, but nevertheless the inference is strong that delusional disorder is not genetically related to schizophrenia. This was a result similar to those of Watt, Hall and Olley (1980) and Kendler and Hays (1981), who did not find an excess of schizophrenia in the relatives of delusional disorder patients. Likewise, the present author (Munro, 1982) in his study of 50 individuals with monosymptomatic hypochondriacal psychosis (i.e. delusional disorder, somatic subtype) could find little evidence of schizophrenia amongst their relatives. Kendler (1982) in a study of demographic factors in delusional disorder, reported that the illness did not appear to resemble closely either schizophrenia or affective illness. A somewhat dissenting opinion is that of Schanda and colleagues (1983), who found more schizophrenics in the relatives of delusional disorder cases, but these workers were utilising a different and more inclusive definition of delusional disorder.

Studies of paranoid schizophrenia are, in general, a little more conclusive. As noted above, Farmer, McGuffin and Gottesman (1987) found fewer cases of schizophrenia in the relatives of paranoid schizophrenics as compared with other schizophrenics, and Kendler and Davis (1981) had earlier noted a similar, though somewhat more tentative, trend. In addition, the latter authors found a tendency for the paranoid type of schizophrenia to breed true in families.

Many descriptions of delusional disorder and of schizophrenia comment on the premorbid personalities of sufferers from these illnesses. Elsewhere in this book (p.13) this writer has referred to this and has pointed out that there may be great difficulty in differentiating retrospectively between premorbid personality and the insidious effects of a slow onset illness (a type of onset which characterizes at least half the cases of delusional disorder). Nevertheless, there remains a strong impression that a considerable number of individuals with 'paranoid' disorders have abnormal personalities predating the start of their psychosis.

It is therefore of interest that there has been a small number of studies on personality patterns among the close relatives of patients with schizophrenia and related illnesses. Kendler and Gruenberg (1982) reported that paranoid personality disorder was relatively frequent in the families of individuals with 'schizophrenic spectrum' conditions. Kendler, Masterson and Ungaro (1984) also noted that schizophrenia-related personality disorders were higher in first-degree relatives of schizophrenics than in those of non-psychiatric controls. In a personal study (Munro, 1982), 10 out of 50 cases were regarded as having longstanding schizoid personality disorders, 1 had histrionic personality features, and 3 had undefined personality disorders – a total of 28 per cent. Thirty per cent of the same group admitted to psychiatric problems in their close relatives and, while details were often missing, the majority of these seemed to have had personality or alcohol-abuse difficulties. In general agreement with this is Winokur's 1985 report on 29 cases of nonhallucinatory delusional disorder patients whose relatives showed an excess of suspicious, secretive or jealous traits and, in some cases, delusions.

In conclusion, therefore, the evidence is scanty, but we seem to have some indication that schizophrenia and paranoid schizophrenia are genetically separate, with a tendency for the latter to follow its own separate genetic line of descent. There is also some agreement that delusional disorder is not a genetic variant of schizophrenia, paranoid schizophrenia or major mood disorder, although there may be a possibility that paranoid and schizoid traits run in the families of delusional disorder patients and are premorbid features in at least a proportion of delusional disorder individuals. Having said this, it has to be emphasized again that the supporting evidence is of the flimsiest and that there is a desperate need for more systematic research in this field.

Organic factors in the aetiology of delusional disorder

As will be evident from other sections of this book, our knowledge of the aetiology of paranoia/delusional disorder is rudimentary and has been enormously hampered by looseness of definition and a tendency, until recently, to lump delusional disorder with schizophrenia. As will be noted, speculative psychoanalytic writings have perhaps given some insights into the delusional content in cases of paranoid disorder but have done nothing to explain the illnesses themselves. German psychiatry has, amongst other background factors, emphasized the role of the 'sensitive' personality, and has claimed that suspiciousness arising in individuals of this type is comprehensible in the light of their attitudes (Kretschmer, 1927), but Fish (1974) and the present author (Munro, 1995) have insisted that a paranoid psychosis is in no way an understandable development of the personality.

Psychological studies (see Chapter 1) have tended to concentrate on the characteristics of delusions or the individuals suffering from them, and clinical psychologists have been active in producing hypotheses about the genesis of delusions (e.g. Maher, 1992; Garety and Hemsley, 1994) but have been unable to produce any really convincing aetiological theories for delusional illnesses. It is this author's belief that the most dramatic results in this field are likely to emerge from neurobiological and neuropathological studies, and already there are fascinating, though tentative, findings available. As Gorman and Cummings (1990) modestly remark, 'Study of organic delusions is in a primitive state', but it is a rapidly developing area of study and already, in one type of delusional disorder, the delusional misidentification syndromes (see Chapter 9) there is good presumptive evidence of underlying brain pathology and even some hints of cerebral localisation.

We have known for many years that, while paranoid disorders often arise idiopathically, a proportion appear to be secondary to other disorders (Cornelius and colleagues, 1991; Tölle, 1993). For example, many of us have seen a situation in which a head injury has caused an equable individual to develop an irritable, over-sensitive personality. We know there is an association between alcoholism and the onset of delusional jealousy (Michael and colleagues, 1995); old age can be associated with the appearance of delusional disorder or late onset schizophrenia, with evidence of associated brain changes; and amphetamine intoxication can produce symptoms apparently typical of paranoid schizophrenia (Connell, 1958; Hall and colleagues, 1988).

As noted in the section on 'late' paraphrenia and schizophrenia of late onset (see Chapter 8), some cases of late onset delusional disorder are associated with noncortical cerebral lesions and Botteron, Figiel and Zorumski (1991) report on three patients with delusional illnesses of old age, all of whom showed caudate abnormalities and two of whom had deep white matter lesions. Feinstein and Ron (1990) studied 65 cases of organic brain syndrome and found that many had presentations which appeared delusional, especially a schizophrenia-like presentation or, to a lesser extent, like mood disorder. Webb (1990) and particularly Gorman and Cummings (1990) have provided excellent reviews of organic delusional syndromes, and have emphasized the extraordinary number of systemic illnesses, toxic disorders and structural brain disorders which may be associated with delusional symptoms and, at times, with actual delusional disorders which nowadays could meet DSMIV or ICD10 criteria.

On a more anecdotal level, other writers have described cocaine-induced paranoia and parasitosis (for example Baker, 1988; Satel and Edell, 1991), monosymptomatic parasitosis associated with ischaemic cerebrovascular disease (Flynn and colleagues, 1989), paranoid psychosis due to AIDS-induced brain damage, and paranoid disorder associated with hyperthyroidism (Steinberg, 1994). The list can be extended enormously.

Gorman and Cummings (1990) suggest that many of the delusional cases of organic origin have common underlying features, particularly temporal lobe or limbic involvement, and they mention studies in which cases of multiple sclerosis, Wernicke's aphasia, epilepsy or Alzheimer's disease have aped delusional disorder and have especially been found to disrupt these brain areas. They also mention the strong possibility of dopamine overactivity being involved in such cases.

One feature which has greatly impressed the present author (Munro, 1982, 1988a) in his own series of cases of monosymptomatic hypochondriacal psychosis (otherwise known as delusional disorder, somatic subtype) is that, whether there appears to be an associated organic aetiological factor or not, the clinical picture and treatment outcome appear to be very much the same. This highlights the artificiality of trying to distinguish between 'organic' and 'functional' disorders when all are, in any case, due to brain dysfunction; the term 'organic' should therefore be restricted to cases where the brain disease is gross and apparent on investigation.

In this writer's series of 50 patients, 16 (32 per cent) admitted to a previous history of serious substance abuse. Twelve individuals gave evidence of a significant cerebral insult at some time in their lives, which might be due to head injury, stroke, diabetic neuropathy or cerebrovascular disease. In total, 20 of the cases could be regarded as having undergone some form of brain damage and the more specific the damage, the earlier did the illness appear to declare itself. Therefore, one could say that 40 per cent of the 50 individuals were suffering from 'secondary' delusional disorder, yet clinically they could not be distinguished from the 60 per cent of 'primary' patients. It is therefore a reasonable contention that organic factors are of great importance in paranoia/delusional disorder. Heredity may play a background role, although as already mentioned, this is speculative on the strength of currently available information, and there is virtually no evidence one way or the other for external stress factors. But there is this highly suggestive evidence that drug and alcohol abuse plus head injury are important predisposing factors, especially in younger males, and equally the ageing brain seems to be of significance, especially in older females. Whether such factors are sufficient in themselves or whether they have to act on a vulnerable substrate in order to evoke paranoia is uncertain. Either way, it has become pedantic and unprofitable to try to distinguish delusional disorder cases as primary or secondary unless, as stated, the organic brain disorder is paramount and the delusional symptoms are clearly a by-product of it.

Delusional disorders – interplay with mood factors

In practice it is not unusual to see delusional or schizophrenic illnesses with significant associated mood symptoms, usually depressive but sometimes manic, and of course cases of depression with delusional features are well documented. This section deals with the ways in which mood features can co-exist with delusional disorder: once again this is not particularly well documented because of the rarity with which delusional disorder was diagnosed until recently, and some inferences have to be drawn from the literature on schizophrenia which is more substantial. The present author has considered this subject in some detail in an earlier publication (Munro, 1988b).

Johnson (1986) notes that the presence of mood symptoms in schizophrenia has been described since the time of Kraepelin and Bleuler. Depression is known to occur in the prodromal phase in some schizophrenics (House, Bostock and Cooper, 1987) but is also recognized in the acute onset phase (Johnson, 1988) and, especially, in the recovery phase. Mayer-Gross (1920) presaged the concept of post-psychotic depression in a classical article and this has been well substantiated subsequently (Mandel and colleagues, 1982). The depressive symptoms which occur within the schizophrenic illness itself may resemble dysphoria (Gabriel, 1987) or major mood disorder (Johnson, 1986).

Post-psychotic depression has been reported as occurring in up to 50 per cent of recovering schizophrenics but 25 per cent is a more usual figure (Mandel and colleagues, 1982). Its aetiology is unclear. Hirsch (1982) and others have advocated the concept of 'revealed depression', suggesting that it is an integral part of the schizophrenic illness which becomes uncovered as the illness improves. Another view is that it is related to the patient's underlying personality or to external stresses to which they become more responsive as the psychosis improves. Increasingly, it seems, the concept of schizoaffective disorder is raised in this context because of the mixture of symptomatologies: this does not carry much credibility (Brockington and Leff, 1979) and elsewhere in this book this writer has emphasized the need to avoid indiscriminate use of this term.

In recent times, the problem of mood disorder occurring in combination with schizophrenia has been made more complex by the effect of neuroleptic drugs both on the patient and on the illness. For example, drug-induced akinesia may look like depression but is likely to respond to antiparkinsonian medication (Van Putten and May, 1978; Johnson, 1981). Also, there has been a tendency to blame neuroleptics for having a depressogenic effect which may occur in some cases but does not explain the great majority of post-psychotic depressions (Johnson, 1986). The present author's speculative view is that major mood disorder is a less disintegrative disorder than schizophrenia. As the latter improves with treatment or by natural remission and as mental functions begin to reintegrate, the patient may then become capable of exhibiting the somewhat higher order symptoms characteristic of depressive disorder, perhaps as a result of some built-in predisposition.

In recent years there has been a small but suggestive number of reports indicating a similar phenomenon in relation to delusional disorders. As indicated, the material is limited because of a lack of extended case series and, until recently, diagnostic accuracy in this area has often been questionable. The author's own series of 50 patients with delusional disorder, somatic subtype (Munro, 1982), all of whom were treated with pimozide, was associated with six cases of severe depression during recovery: although many of the patients had been unhappy or dejected as a result of their illness, none had a previous history of major mood disorder. It was concluded that the post-psychotic depression was not a side effect of the medication, and treatment was usually successful when adequate dosages of antidepressant were added to the pimozide regime.

Interestingly, although a few of these patients had been treated already with other neuroleptics with no success, some did report a slight lessening of their delusional preoccupation while previously on a tricyclic antidepressant by itself. This observation has been replicated by others, for example Cashman and Pollock (1983), who described a partial response in a case of delusional disorder, somatic subtype, with imipramine. Chiu, McFarlane and Dobson (1990) report on four cases of monodelusional psychosis associated with depression which improved markedly on a combination of pimozide and clomipramine.

Other authors have commented on a small number of cases of paranoid disorder (whose provenance is not always totally clear) which have done particularly well with a variety of antidepressants such as doxepin and imipramine (Brotman and Jenike, 1984), tricyclics and phenelzine (Akiskal and colleagues, 1983), and trazodone (Sheehy, 1983). Singh and Maguire (1984) described a schizophrenic who developed manic symptoms on pipotiazine palmitate and, on the other hand, there is a single case report of an individual apparently precipitated into a monodelusional disorder by the use of the monoamine oxidase inhibitor, phenelzine (Liebowitz, Nuetzel and Bowser, 1978).

Delusional and mood disorders are separate illnesses with their own natural histories and treatment responses, but there is a relationship, albeit a subtle and complex one, between them. The questions raised by this are thoughtfully considered in an article by Ross, Siddiqui and Matas (1987). Jørgensen (1989) has described a series of cases in which the differentiation between delusional and mood illnesses is, at times, impossible; and Fry (1978) noted that episodic illness which is apparently delusional may be the result of an underlying bipolar mood disorder. Many of us have seen cases in which a seeming major mood disorder gradually deteriorated into schizophrenia or delusional disorder and Logsdail (1984) describes three cases of such a phenomenon.

Delusional disorder: a brief commentary on psychodynamic contributions

Much of the psychoanalytic literature or its derivatives continue to talk in terms of 'paranoia' (for example, Oldham and Bone, 1994) and often does not make it clear whether a trait, a personality disorder, a symptom or a syndrome is under consideration. Freud, of course, presented his theories of paranoia (by which he usually meant the delusional illness) and these are still acknowledged with respect by many psychodynamic therapists. He emphasized libidinal processes, proposing that paranoia was a regression from the homosexual phase of psychosexual development to a fixation at the primary narcissistic phase. Homosexual love, which is unacceptable to the individual, is transformed by projection into suspiciousness and rejection (Freud, 1958a, b). The Freudian concept of repressed homosexuality has not met with total acceptance and Aronson (1989) notes that later psychoanalysts found evidence of it only in a minority of paranoiac patients. Ovesey (1954, 1955) spoke of a 'pseudohomosexual' conflict in males who inhibit their aggressiveness as a result of childhood power struggles with their parents.

Klein (1957) stated that homosexual love was indeed an important element in paranoia but behind it was profound hatred and a wish by the infant to destroy the devouring parent. In her theory, paranoia was a fixation at the paranoid–schizoid position, which she believed to occur between six and nine months in the developing infant. Also, the child is envious of other women who represent the mother's breast and this envy is a powerful motivation towards paranoia.

Many theories invoke narcissistic elements in the aetiology of paranoia. Freud considered that hypochondriasis resulted from a turning of the libido from external objects on to the self, with subsequent change of the excessive narcissistic investment in body organs into physical symptoms. Kohut (1977) regards narcissism as an essential driving force in the psychic economy and presents paranoia as due to empathic failures and narcissistic injuries by parents which cause defective formation of the developing self.

There are many more generalised suggestions about paranoia. For example, Fenichel (1945) saw paranoid delusions as a relief by way of projection from shame, guilt and inadequacy generated by an excessively potent superego. Sullivan (1953) thought that persecutory and grandiose ideas overcome inferiority and weakness and implied that, for some individuals, paranoia was a more comfortable state than a tortured sanity; one can only say he must have been very fortunate if he observed many contented paranoiacs. Aronson (1989) described the paranoid as living in a state of continually threatened autonomy, a much more insightful view of the distress suffered by most delusional disorder patients.

In some psychodynamic theories, paranoia and depression are linked. As already indicated, there do seem to be points of contact between delusional and mood disorders but one cannot venture to suggest whether there is an aetiological connection. Salzman (1960), however, baldly states that paranoia is a response to underlying depression; Meissner (1978) says that 'paranoid patients can only relinquish their paranoid stance at the risk of encountering a severe depression'; and Millar (1989) avers that the 'paranoid cycle' is related to a fluctuation in the state of the 'omnipotence illusion' (the adult version of the omnipotence phase of the young child). This last author believes that depression is 'omnipotence lost' and paranoia is 'omnipotence threatened'.

A recurring theme is that of inadequacy counteracted by the aggressiveness of paranoia (Kohut, 1977) and of aggressiveness projected on to external objects who then become persecutors (Hesselbach, 1962).

Much of the psychoanalytic and subsequent psychodynamic literature concentrates on the persecutory type of paranoia (often, it seems, because it is assumed that that is virtually the only type of delusional content found in the illness). However, grandiosity as a defence against inadequacy is mentioned (Millar, 1989) and mention was made above to theories regarding somatic/hypochondriacal delusions. There is even a reference to psychodynamic aspects of infestation delusions (Torch and Bishop, 1981) in which these phenomena are referred to unsatisfied dependency needs, domination by significant others and feelings of inadequacy and worthlessness.

Morbid jealousy has been similarly dissected and has been linked to masturbatory fantasies with masochistic and narcissistic elements (Coen, 1987), and to sadistic and exhibitionistic traits (Freeman, 1990). Klein's (1957) previously noted views on envy are often quoted in this context.

In summary, this is admittedly an abbreviated and superficial review of psychodynamic views on paranoid illnesses. The psychoanalytic reader will be utterly dissatisfied with the sketchiness of the approach, but it would go against the principle on which this book is designed to elaborate further, or appear to give undue credence to speculative theories on paranoia. In our current state of development in psychiatry it is essential that we eschew our long-established tendencies to theorise rather than experiment and to explain rather than correlate.

Science is beginning to make the most tentative of inroads in dispelling our ignorance about delusions and delusional disorders and is doing this by dint of careful observation and cautious juxtaposition of data. Psychodynamic theories were exciting when other methodologies were unavailable. Nowadays we can only regard as bathetic many of the statements we read in the psychodynamic literature, old or new: for example, take Freud's aphorism, 'People become paranoiac over things that they cannot put up with, provided that they possess the peculiar psychical disposition for it'. An equally profound statement might be that an animal will escape from its stalker by flying over a wall, provided it is a bird.

This is not to be facetious. Psychoanalysis has indeed provided many therapists with a paradigm by which they can approach the treatment of certain patients. It has rarely provided a datum which reliably informs us about the origin of delusions or about the aetiology of delusional disorders. The reader should not be persuaded otherwise.

Conclusion

Kraepelin (1921), almost a century ago, clearly differentiated between mood disorders, delusional disorders, schizophrenia and organic brain disorders, although he recognized that all of these illnesses had certain features in common, including delusions. Nevertheless, he emphasized their individually distinctive characteristics as well as their different natural histories and outcomes. To an increasing extent we can add nowadays the differential responses to specific treatments. For many years after his time, the nosological scene in psychiatry was a desert, especially in the United States where, in many centres, diagnostic precision was largely swept away and virtually everything 'bizarre' became schizophrenic. Paranoia/delusional disorder, because of a superficial resemblance to schizophrenia, was confused with that illness and psychiatrists mostly ceased to be aware of it, although they still used terms like 'paranoia' and 'paranoid' without bothering to define them.

Schizophrenia, as an overall group, is breaking up and delusional disorder is one of the first disorders to depart from an over-inclusive category. It is rewarding to see that the conceptualization and description of delusional disorder are now being advanced and it is safe to say that there is a fruitful field of research here for the coming generation.

Let us now consider each of the subtypes of delusional disorder in more detail.

References

Akiskal, H.S., Arana, G.W., Baldessarini, R.J. andBarreira, P.J. (1983). A clinical report of thymoleptic-responsive atypical paranoid psychoses. *Am. J. Psychiat.* **140**: 1187–1190.

Aronson, T.A. (1989). Paranoia and narcissism in psychoanalytic theory. *Psychoanalyt. Rev.* **76**: 329–351.

Axelson, R. and Wahlström, J. (1984). Chromosome aberrations in patients with paranoid psychosis. *Hereditas* **100**: 29–31.

Baker, F.M. (1988). Cocaine psychosis. *J. Nat. Med. Ass.* **81**:987–1000.

Berner, P. (1965). *Das Paranoische Syndrom.* Berlin: Springer.

Botteron, K., Figiel, G.S. and Zorumski, C.F. (1991). Electroconvulsive therapy in patients with late-onset psychosis and structured brain changes. *J. Geriat. Psychiat. Neurol.* **4**: 44–47.

Brockington, I .F. and Leff, J.P. (1979). Schizoaffective psychosis: definitions and incidence. *Psychol. Med.* **9**: 91–99.

Brotman, A.W. and Jenike, M.A. (1984). Monosymptomatic hypochondriasis treated with tricyclic antidepressants. *Am. J. Psychiat* **141**: 1608–1609.

Cashman, F.E. and Pollock, B. (1983). Treatment of monosymptomatic hypochondriacal psychosis with imipramine. *Can. J. Psychiat.* **28**: 85 (letter).

Chiu, S., McFarlane, A.H. and Dobson, N. (1990). The treatment of monodelusional psychosis associated with depression. *Br. J. Psychiat.* **156**: 112–115.

Coen, S.J. (1987). Pathological jealousy. *Int. J. Psycho-Anal.* **68**: 99–108.

Connell, P.H. (1958). *Amphetamine Psychosis.* Maudsley Monograph No. 5. London: Chapman & Hall.

Cooper, A.F., Curry, A.R. and Kay, D.W.K. (1974). Hearing loss in paranoid and affective psychoses of the elderly. *Lancet* **2**: 851–854.

Cornelius, J.R., Day, N.L., Fabrega, H., Mezzich, J., Cornelius, M.D. and Ulrich, R.F. (1991). Characterizing organic delusional syndrome. *Arch. Gen. Psychiat.* **48**: 749–753.

Diagnostic and Statistical Manual of Mental Disorders, 3rd edn revised (DSMIIIR) (1987). Washington, DC: American Psychiatric Association.

Diagnostic and Statistical Manual of Mental Disorders, 4th edn (DSMIV) (1994) Washington, DC: American Psychiatric Association.

Farmer, A.E., McGuffin, P. and Gottesman, I.I. (1987). Searching for the split in schizophrenia: a twin study perspective. *Psychiat. Res.* **13**: 109–118.

Feinstein, A. and Ron, M.A. (1990). Psychosis associated with demonstrable brain disease. *Psychol. Med.* **20**: 793–803.

Fenichel, O. (1945). *The Psychoanalytic Theory of Neurosis.* New York: Norton.

Fish, F.J. (1974). *Clinical Psychopathology*, ed. M. J. Hamilton. Bristol: John Wright & Sons.

Flaum, M., Arndt, S. and Andreasen, N.C. (1991). The reliability of 'bizarre' delusions. *Compr. Psychiat.* **32**: 59–65.

Flynn, F.G., Cummings, J.L., Scheibel, J. and Wirshing, W. (1989). Monosymptomatic delusions of parasitosis associated with ischemic cerebrovascular disease. *J. Geriat. Psychiat. Neurol.* **2**: 134–139.

Freeman, T. (1990). Psychoanalytical aspects of morbid jealousy in women. *Br. J. Psychiat.* **156**: 68–72.

Freud, S. (1958a). *Extracts from the Fliess Papers*, standard edn, Vol. 1, pp. 173–280. London: Hogarth Press.

Freud, S. (1958b). *The Case of Schreber* (Complete Works), Vol. 12, ed. by J. Strachey. London: Hogarth Press.

Fry, W.F. (1978). Paranoid episodes in manic–depressive psychoses. *Am. J. Psychiat.* **135**: 974–976.

Gabriel, E. (1987). Dysphoric mood in paranoid psychoses. *Psychopathology* **20**: 101–106.

Garety, P. A. and Hemsley, D. R. (1994) *Delusions: Investigations into the Psychology of Delusional Reasoning*. Maudsley Monograph No. 36. Oxford: Oxford University Press.

Gloag, D. (1980). Noise: hearing loss and psychological effects. *Br. Med. J.* **281**: 1325–1327.

Goldstein, R.L. (1987). Litigious paranoids and the legal system:the role of the forensic psychiatrist. *J. Forens. Sci. (JFSCA)*, **32**: 1009–1115.

Gorman, D.G. and Cummings, J.L. (1990). Organic delusional syndrome. *Sem. Neurol.* **10**: 229–238.

Guensberger, E., Fleischer, J. and Sipkovska, E. (1977). On the psychopathology of paranoid psychosis in the blind. *Cesk. Psychiat.* **73**: 291–296.

Hall, R.C.W., Popkin, M.K., Beresford, T.P. and Hall, A.K. (1988). Amphetamine psychosis: clinical presentations and differential diagnosis. *Psychiat. Med.* **6**: 73–79.

Hawes, M.J. and Bible, H.H. (1990). The paranoid patient: surgeon beware! *Ophthal. Plas. Reconstr. Surg.* **6**: 225–227.

Hesselbach, C.F. (1962). Superego regression in paranoia. *Psychoanalyt. Q.* **31**: 341–350.

Hirsch, S. (1982). Depression 'revealed' in schizophrenia. *Br. J. Psychiat.* **140**: 421–424.

House, A., Bostock, J. and Cooper, J. (1987). Depressive syndromes in the year following onset of a first schizophrenic illness. *Br. J. Psychiat.* **151**: 773–779.

Jaspers, K. (1963). *General Psychopathology*, transl. by J. Hoenig and M. Hamilton. Manchester: University of Manchester Press.

Johnson, D.A.W. (1981). Studies of depressive symptoms in schizophrenia. *Br. J. Psychiat.* **139**: 89–101.

Johnson, D.A.W. (1986). Depressive symptoms in schizophrenia: some observations on the frequency, morbidity and possible causes. In *Contemporary Issues of Schizophrenia*, ed. A. Kerr and P. Snaith. London: Gaskell.

Johnson, D.A.W. (1988). The significance of depression in the prediction of relapse in chronic schizophrenia. *Br. J. Psychiat.* **152**: 320–323.

Jørgensen, P. (1989). Classification and outcome in nonschizophrenic, nonaffective delusional psychoses. *Psychopathol.* **22**: 198–201.

Kay, D.W.K. and Roth, M. (1961). Factors in schizophrenia of old age. *J. Ment. Sci.* **107**: 649–686.

Kendler, K.S. (1982). Demography of paranoid psychosis (delusional disorder): a review and comparison with schizophrenia and affective illness. *Arch. Gen. Psychiat.* **39**: 890–902.

Kendler, K.S. (1987). Paranoid disorders in DSMIII, a critical review. In *Diagnosis and Classification in Psychiatry*, ed. G. L. Tischler. Cambridge: Cambridge University Press.

Kendler, K.S. and Davis, K.L. (1981). The genetics and biochemistry of paranoid schizophrenia and other paranoid psychoses. *Schizophr. Bull.* **7**: 689–709.

Kendler, K.S. and Gruenberg, A.M. (1982). Genetic relationship between paranoid personality disorder and the 'schizophrenic spectrum' disorders. *Am. J. Psychiat.* **139**:1185–1186.

Kendler, K.S. and Hays, P. (1981). Paranoid psychosis (delusional disorder) and schizophrenia: a family history study. *Arch. Gen. Psychiat.* **38**: 547–551.

Kendler, K.S., Masterson, C.C. and Ungaro, R. (1984). A family history study of schizophrenia-related personality disorders. *Am. J. Psychiat.* **141**: 424–427.

Klein, M. (1957). Envy and gratitude. In *The Writings of Melanie Klein*, vol. 3, pp. 176–235. London: Hogarth Press.

Kohut, H. (1977). *The Restoration of the Self.* New York: International Universities.

Kraepelin, E. (1921). *Manic Depressive Insanity and Paranoia.* Transl. by R. M. Barclay. (1976). New York: Arno Press.

Kretschmer, E. (1927). *Der sensitive Berziehungswahn*, 2nd edn. Berlin: Springer.

Liebowitz, M.R., Nuetzel, E.J. and Bowser, A.E. (1978). Phenelzine and delusions of parasitosis: a case report. *Am. J. Psychiat.* **135**: 1565–1566.

Lipowski, Z.J. (1980). *Delirium*, pp. 74–75. Springfield, Ill.: Charles C. Thomas.

Logsdail, S. (1984). Affective illness changing to paranoid state. Report on three elderly patients. *Br. J. Psychiat.* **144**: 209–210.

Maher, B.A. (1992). Delusions: contemporary etiological hypotheses. *Psychiatr. Ann.* **22**: 260–268.

Mandel, M.R., Severe, J.B., Schooler, N.R., Gelenberg, A.J. and Mieske, M. (1982). Development and prediction of postpsychotic depression in neuroleptic-treated schizophrenics. *Arch. Gen. Psychiat* **39**: 197–203.

Mayer-Gross, W. (1920). Über die stellungsnahme auf abgelanfench akuten psychosen. *Ztsch. ges. Neurol. Psychiat.* **60**: 160–212.

Meissner, W.W. (1978). *The Paranoid Process.* New York: Jason Aronson.

Michael, A., Mirza, S., Mirza, K.A.H., Babu, V.S. and Vithayathil, E. (1995). Morbid jealousy in alcoholism. *Br. J. Psychiat.* **167**: 668–672.

Millar, T.P. (1989). Childhood precursors of the paranoid–depressive disorder. *Perspect. Biol. Med.* **32**: 539–546.

Mojtabai, R. and Nicholson, R.A. (1995). Interrater reliability of ratings of delusions and bizarre delusions. *Am. J. Psychiat.* **152**: 1804–1806.

Munro, A. (1982). *Delusional Hypochondriasis.* Clarke Institute of Psychiatry Monograph Series No. 5. Toronto: Clarke Institute of Psychiatry.

Munro, A. (1988a). Delusional (paranoid) disorders: etiologic and taxonomic considerations. I: The possible significance of organic brain factors in etiology of delusional disorders. *Can. J. Psychiat.* **33**: 171–174.

Munro, A. (1988b). Delusional (paranoid) disorders: etiologic and taxonomic considerations. II: A possible relationship between delusional and affective disorders. *Can. J. Psychiat.* **33**:175–178.

Munro, A. (1992). Psychiatric disorders characterized by delusions: treatment in relation to specific types. *Psychiat. Ann.* **22**: 232–240.

Munro, A. (1995). The classification of delusional disorders. *Psychiat. Clin. N.*

Am. **18**: 199–212.

Oldham, J.M. and Bone, S. (1994). *Paranoia: New Psychoanalytic Perspectives.* Madison and Connecticut: International Universities Press.

Ovesey, L. (1954). The homosexual conflict: an adaptational analysis. *Psychiatry* **17**: 243–250.

Ovesey, L. (1955). Pseudohomosexuality, the paranoid mechanism and paranoia. *Psychiatry* **18**: 163–173.

Retterstøl, N. (1966). *Paranoid and Paranoiac Psychoses.* Springfield, Ill.: Charles C. Thomas.

Ross, C.A., Siddiqui, A.R. and Matas, M. (1987). DSMIII: problems in diagnosis of paranoia and obsessive–compulsive disorder. *Can. J. Psychiat.* **32**: 146–148.

Rowlands, M.W.D. (1988). Psychiatric and legal aspects of persistent litigation. *Br. J. Psychiat.* **153**: 317–323.

Salzman, O. (1960). Paranoid state: theory and therapy. *Arch. Gen. Psychiat.* **2**: 679–693.

Satel, S.L. and Edell, W.S. (1991). Cocaine-induced paranoia and psychosis-proneness. *Am. J. Psychiat.* **148**: 1708–1711.

Schanda, H., Berner, P., Gabriel, E., Kronberger, M.L. and Kufferle, B. (1983). The genetics of delusional psychoses. *Schizophr. Bull.* **9**: 563–570.

Sheehy, M. (1983). Successful treatment of paranoia with trazodone. *Am. J. Psychiat.* **140**: 945 (letter).

Singh, A.N. and Maguire, J. (1984). Pipothiazine palmitate induced mania. *Br. Med. J.* **189**: 734 (letter).

Steinberg, P.I. (1994). A case of paranoid disorder associated with hyperthyroidism. *Can. J. Psychiat.* **39**: 153–156.

Sullivan, H.S. (1953). *Conceptions of Modern Psychiatry.* New York: Norton.

Thomas, A.J. (1981). Acquired deafness and mental health. *Br. J. Med. Psychol.* **54**: 219–229.

Tölle, R. (1993). Somatopsychic aspects of paranoia. *Psychopathology* **26**: 127–137.

Torch, E.M. and Bishop, E.R. (1981). Delusions of parasitosis: psychotherapeutic engagement. *Am. J. Psychother.* **35**: 101–106.

Van Putten, T. and May, P.R.A. (1978). 'Akinetic depression' in schizophrenia. *Arch. Gen. Psychiat.* **35**: 1101–1107.

Watt, J.A.G. (1985). Hearing and premorbid personality in paranoid states. *Am. J. Psychiat.* **142**: 1453–1455.

Watt, J.A.G., Hall, D.J. and Olley, P.C. (1980). Paranoid states of middle life. Familial occurrence and relationship to schizophrenia. *Acta Psychiat. Scand.* **61**: 413–426.

Webb, W. (1990). Paranoid conditions seen in psychiatric medicine. *Psychiat. Med.* **8**: 37–48.

Zona, M.A., Sharma, K.K. and Lane, J. (1993). A comparative study of erotomanic and obsessional subjects in a forensic sample. *J. Forens. Sci. (JFSCA)* **38**: 894–903.

3

Delusional disorder, somatic subtype

In this chapter we shall first consider some general aspects of health concern, somatization and hypochondriasis, and then look at relevant areas concerning body image and its disorders. Thereafter we will look at the overall features of delusional disorder of the somatic subtype, then go on to some of the more important specific hypochondriacal delusional presentations which we are likely to encounter.

Somatization and hypochondriasis (Munro, 1988; Kellner, 1992; Warwick and colleagues, 1996)

Modern society, especially in developed countries, is preoccupied with health concerns such as diet, exercise, the need for a clean environment, and the avoidance of toxic substances. While all of this is positive, it is unfortunate that people who are over-concerned with their health are likely to be made excessively anxious, especially as a result of all the media material on health-related subjects which have become so commonplace.

Health concern has two outstanding aspects, the first being a persistent preoccupation with the body and its functions, and the second a persistent concern with health matters. These are quite consistent with normal mental health and motivate people towards positive living styles. Unhappily, some individuals move on to *pathological self-concern* in which there is constant fear of physical symptoms, with over-awareness of physiological signals or exaggeration of slight aches. From there, another sub-group may develop actual *hypochondriasis* in which there is a constant conviction of being ill, misinterpretation of minor symptoms as actual illness, and resistance to reassurance that no serious disorder is present.

Each of these stages represents degrees of severity in the *somatizing* (or *hypochondriacal*) *individual* (Lipowski, 1988; Purcell, 1991), someone who tends to express psychological conflict or actual psychiatric illness as complaints of physical illness. The somatiser exhibits a marked somatic style, partially due to hypochondriasis and partially the result of an inability to express emotions in psychological terms (a phenomenon known as alexithymia) (Sifneos, 1973). In addition, patients often show an unreasonable fear of disease (*disease phobia*) and an over-readiness to believe that they are actually ill (*disease conviction*). Some people also display a degree of body image disturbance which can take two principal forms: The first is a dysmorphic belief in which the individual is unreasonably convinced that the body is malformed in some way, and, as will be seen, this can take a delusional form in some patients; the second is coenaesthesiopathy where there is misinterpretation of bodily sensations so that an itch, a slight pain or profuse sweating may be regarded as evidence of serious pathology, which may sometimes be the starting point for a delusion of infestation (Brink and colleagues, 1979).

Characteristics of the somatizing patient (Katon and colleagues, 1991)

The individual has physical symptoms typical of somatic illness with no convincing evidence of underlying physical disease or of a physiological mechanism which could explain the symptoms. If an actual physical disorder is present, it is not sufficient to explain the complaint. In addition, significant emotional conflicts or a diagnosable psychiatric illness are found to be present, and a 'psychological gain' motivation is not infrequent.

Complaints often seem reasonable at first, but repetitive pursuit of medical care and insistent complaining associated with the inability to be reassured should soon make the physician aware that the complaining is not reasonable at all. It becomes obvious that the person has adopted a sick role and is determined to cling to his 'illness'.

It has to be emphasized that it is not sufficient to diagnose a hypochondriacal disorder just because no accompanying physical pathology has been found: it must be accompanied by a convincing psychiatric element. We must also be aware that certain truly physical disorders are sometimes mistaken for hypochondriasis, especially in their early stages, and these include multiple sclerosis, systemic lupus erythematosus, myasthenia gravis and porphyria.

Psychiatric illnesses associated with severe somatization

Hypochondriasis may be a personality trait without much other evidence of psychopathology, but it may also be an accompaniment of many psychiatric conditions. Any of the following may be associated with marked hypochondriasis and physical complaining:

(1) Somatoform disorders
(2) Delusional disorder of the somatic subtype, also known as mono-symptomatic hypochondriacal psychosis, or MHP
(3) Anxiety disorder
(4) Depressive disorder
(5) Obsessive–compulsive disorder
(6) Schizophrenia
(7) Various personality disorders
(8) Dementia, especially in its earlier stages.

All of these are important but, in the present context, it is the hypochondriasis of delusional disorder which will shortly be considered in detail. Others from the above list, especially somatoform disorder and obsessive–compulsive disorder, will be mentioned elsewhere (see Chapter 12). Before moving to the various forms of the delusional disorder, let us briefly consider some points concerning the recognition of somatizing illnesses.

The general recognition of somatizing patients

(1) First, be aware that hypochondriasis in general is very common indeed (Barsky and colleagues, 1990), and that delusional hypochondriasis is certainly not rare (Munro, 1982).
(2) When carrying out a physical examination always take time to do a brief review of the patient's mental state.
(3) Obtain a confirmatory history but be aware of *folie à deux* in, especially, delusional disorder cases: in this situation one may obtain totally false but convincing confirmation. Also, obtain access to previous records.
(4) Note any marked discrepancy between complaint, history and findings.
(5) Many hypochondriacal patients are unduly importunate and persistent.
(6) If physical pathology is actually present, it is usually irrelevant.
(7) Look for evidence of multiple operations, especially in younger patients.

(8) In some, but far from all, cases there may be drug-seeking.

(9) Often, incessant new complaints and failure to respond to reassurance are suggestive.

(10) Many hypochondriacs attend multiple physicians, both in series and in parallel.

(11) Sometimes there is a psychological gain motive but this is usually not evident in delusional disorder.

(12) Hypochondriacal cases often seem to be getting out of the physician's control.

(13) A multitude of investigations and treatments only seem to make the complaining worse.

Body image and its disorders

Once more we find a field bedevilled by confusing terminology, and Cumming (1988) comments on the interchangeable use of terms like body schema, body experience, body image, body concept, somatopsyche, image of the body ego, and body awareness. He suggests that 'body schema' should be used to denote the individual's awareness of the spatial characteristics of his or her own body, and 'body experience' to denote body schema plus associated psychological, situational, emotional and intentional factors. Cumming notes that the parietal lobes of the cerebrum play a major part in underpinning the normal body schema, with important contributions from the somatoaesthetic afferent system and the thalamus, and he succinctly reviews the neurobiology and neuropathology of the body schema with clinical illustrations of how it may become perverted in a number of ways.

Pruzinsky (1990) uses the alternative term 'body image' and says that much of the recent work on the subject has been done in relation to eating disorders. In recent years there has also been a considerable interest in body dysmorphic disorder (see Chapter 12). He cites research on other areas, including hypochondriasis, somatic delusions, trans-sexualism, self-mutilation, etc., but emphasizes the difficulty of collating these materials because they are scattered across several disciplines and literatures (a problem already noted as being shared by the delusional disorders as a whole).

Body image is not simply appearance but can incorporate awareness of strength, body size, the degree of masculinity or femininity, one's experience of one's body boundaries, the overall level of body security, and feelings about emotional arousal. All of these are part of a permanent but somewhat vague perception that each individual has of his or her body. A person with a relatively secure body image/body schema will have a degree of resilience in dealing with changes to it due to illness, ageing, injury and so on and will not usually display excessive health concern. On the other hand, vulnerable individuals may be constantly aware of some deficiency, real or imagined, in the body schema which can cause considerable distress and a prolonged search for 'wholeness'. The nature of that search will determine the form that the search will take. Somatic delusions can arise in a number of psychiatric disorders, including delusional disorder, and represent a severe distortion of the body schema and a distorted attempt to obtain restitution, usually by seeking totally inappropriate treatment.

Pruzinsky and Cash (1990) remark that body image remains rather elusive because it means different things to different people and also because it is not a static quality. It is multifaceted, intertwined with other feelings and perceptions of self, and heavily socially determined. A fascinating and detailed account of body image theory and research is presented in Cash and Pruzinsky's volume on body image (1990).

Delusional disorder, somatic subtype: general concerns

In delusional disorder of the somatic subtype we see a variety of alterations in body schema. As has been noted elsewhere, it is interesting that there seem to be certain themes which predominate, such as distortions of skin perception in delusional parasitosis, in body shape with the dysmorphic delusions, in weight perception in some cases of anorexia nervosa, of awareness of body odour in smell delusions, of facial and dental features, and in delusions of having a profound disease, such as AIDS. There are a number of small and separate literatures describing abnormalities of these types and some of these will shortly be described.

When diagnosing delusional disorder with a somatic complaint, the case should be designated 'delusional disorder, somatic subtype, characterized by a dysmorphic delusion/delusion of disease, etc.', with a description thereafter of the aspect of body structure or function which is involved.

It is ironic that, in Kraepelin's day, although paranoia was so well recognized, a hypochondriacal form was not accepted (see below). In the past 25 years, an increasing amount of information has led to the recognition of just such a disorder and it is now an official subtype of delusional disorder in DSMIV (1994) and ICD10 (1992–93). Not only that, but the relatively intense interest in this particular subtype has led to a re-formulation of the whole paranoia concept and has been partly responsible for the latter's revival under its new title of delusional disorder.

In some ways, therefore, the somatic subtype of delusional disorder is the most clearly described, and has accumulated the most voluminous recent literature on phenomenology and treatment. It is also a disorder which arouses interest amongst medical specialists other than psychiatrists since the cases initially present to them and almost invariably cause considerable problems in diagnosis and management. The discovery that these cases have a psychiatric provenance and that they may be susceptible to treatment is good news to other physicians who are usually very happy to have a psychiatrist help them with management.

The result is that the somatic subtype can be discussed more fully in the light of current knowledge than is possible with other subtypes, where information is of the more traditional type and where fewer series and fewer treatment outcomes have been reported. This may make it seem that cases of the somatic subtype are more numerous or more important than the others, but this is by no means necessarily so. It is very likely that erotomania, jealousy and persecutory delusional disorders are much more common than we know and, as will be seen in other chapters, can cause just as much distress among patients, relatives and therapists as do the somatic forms. There is a pressing need for more recognition of these other subtypes and for systematic work on their treatment.

In the meantime, we have to use the modern information we have on the somatic subtype to flesh out our paradigm of delusional disorder as a whole. This is better than no information at all, but demands a certain caution in interpreting data on the nonsomatic subtypes. What is interesting and hopeful is that very little of what has been noted regarding delusional disorder in modern times seriously contradicts the descriptions from nearly a century ago.

Difficulties in nomenclature

Once more we see a welter of varying terminologies, lack of communication between disciplines, and a dispersal of information through different literatures. Nowadays, when a case with somatic delusions is compared with the other subtypes of paranoia/delusional disorder, we must appreciate that all of these forms closely resemble each other, apart from the content of the delusional system. Until recently this perception was not the case.

Kraepelin's delineation of paranoia remains our lodestone and he clearly described three subtypes whose delusional contents consisted of erotomania, paranoid jealousy and megalomania. He wrote in 1921 that

... a hypochondriacal form is frequently described as another kind of paranoid delusion with depressive colouring. It is certain that hypochondriacal delusions are frequently expressed by paranoiacs. Nevertheless, I have not found it possible in careful sifting of my experiences to find an indubitable case of paranoia characterized only, or at least predominantly, by this kind of delusion. I think therefore that I would meantime abstain from the delimitation of a hypochondriacal paranoia.

This disclaimer may have discouraged others from accepting that the hypochondriacal form not only existed but was well recognized by physicians other than psychiatrists. It is becoming fashionable nowadays for patients to complain of psychological symptoms, but in Kraepelin's time the hypochondriacal individual had little option but to express his or her mental distress in physical terms in order to gain attention. Perhaps if consultation–liaison psychiatry had existed then, psychiatrists might have appreciated much better that, among the mass of patients with hypochondriacal concerns, there were a not inconsiderable number of presentations typical of delusional disorder.

Despite the flourishing of 'psychosomatic' concepts in the mid-twentieth century, there was little or no contribution to the field of somatic overconcerns in delusional disorder until a Swedish psychiatrist, Ekbom (1938) published his pioneering work on presenile infestation delusions, based on seven cases, in some of which the presentation appeared to be monodelusional in nature. His description became identified with that of 'monosymptomatic hypochondriacal psychosis', a concept which was largely restricted to the German and Scandinavian psychiatric communities, and which allowed for a variety of aetiologies and diagnoses, provided the principal symptom was a somatic delusion. Skott (1978), also from Sweden, published an interesting monograph, describing her own cases of delusional parasitosis, and endorsing Ekbom's view of the heterogeneity of the condition.

Both Ekbom and Skott were perfectly correct about this mixture of diagnoses. They were interested in patients who had delusions in which they (the patients) were convinced that they had insects on or under their skin which no one else could detect – a disorder about which dermatologists had long been aware. And, indeed, if one collects a series of cases defined entirely by that delusional content, one will find that within it there are patients with delusional disorder, schizophrenia, major depression, early dementia and other severe mental illnesses.

As described in Chapter 1, the present author became aware of cases that had a hypochondriacal delusional content in which one symptom predominated over the others. In some patients this was a conviction of insect infestation but in other individuals the delusion concerned physical appearance, giving off a foul smell or some other complaint. The striking thing was that, although the complaint might vary so much, the form of the illness was remarkably similar from case to case. A series based on that monodelusional form was gathered and it was possible to demonstrate that the varying presentations appear to be one and the same illness. The term 'monosymptomatic hypochondriacal psychosis' (MHP) was employed to describe the group.

In 1987, when DSMIIIR appeared and the concept of paranoia was revived but renamed delusional disorder, MHP was recognized as the somatic subtype of this and, following the principle suggested above, delusional disorder was seen as a unitary entity but with subtypes described according to the main delusional content. Hence, we now have jealousy, erotomanic, somatic, persecutory and grandiose subtypes. As will shortly be noted, within the somatic subtype there are a number of themes: so long as the description of the overall illness is that of paranoia/delusional disorder, then that is the basic diagnosis.

With DSMIIIR and DSMIV there is a relatively straightforward exposition of this stance, now confirmed by ICD10. Nevertheless, as already noted, terminology is a serious problem and the area of dermatological delusions is particularly striking with regard to misleading jargons, as we shall now see.

Psychiatrists have been largely ignorant of MHP/delusional disorder, somatic subtype, until relatively recently, and descriptions of different case types have come to us largely from nonpsychiatric sources. Of these, the dermatological literature is the best conceptualised, but so many different terms and formulations have been used even there, that it is often very difficult to be sure what is actually being described. Here are some examples, specifically from dermatology, to illustrate the problems we face:

(1) Berrios (1982) lists the following synonyms for delusional parasitosis:acarophobia, *le délire dermatozoaire, l'hallucinose tactile chronique, parasitoses délirantes*, Chronische Taktile Dermatozoenhallucinose, Dermatozoenwahn, *neurodermies parasitophobiques*, delusory parasitosis, parasitophobia, and dermatophobia – not to mention chronic tactile hallucinosis (Lynch, 1993), *délires de zoopathie externe* (de

Leon, Bott and Simpson, 1989), phantom biters (Edwards, 1977), cutaneous parasitosis (Alexander, 1984), and delusions of infestation (Skott, 1978), etc.

(2) Some cases of trichotillomania (pathological hair-pulling) and onychotillomania (excessive nail-pulling) are associated with delusional beliefs (Dean and colleagues, 1992; Stein and Hollander, 1992; Tanquary, Lynch and Masand, 1992).

(3) 'Cocaine bugs', the delusion of insects crawling over the skin, associated with the sensory abnormality known as 'formication' is a layman's term but a well-known symptom in relation to cocaine and other addictions (Elpern, 1988; Marschall, Dolezal and Cohen, 1991).

(4) Chronic cutaneous dysaesthesia syndrome (Koblenzer and Bostrom, 1994) may occasionally be a delusional disorder.

(5) Bromosis, or delusions of bromosis (Malasi, and colleagues, 1990) (also known as olfactory reference syndrome) – a conviction of giving off an offensive body odour, sometimes attributed to excessive or abnormal sweat, and occasionally seen by dermatologists.

(6) Cases regarded as 'dermatitis artefacta' (Murray, Ross and Murray, 1987) or 'neurotic excoriations' (van Moffaert, 1992) may sometimes be due to infestation delusions complicated by constant scratching or gouging to get rid of the 'parasites'.

All of the above are in addition to other genuine dermatological disorders which are believed to have emotional background factors (van Moffaert, 1992).

No doubt a similar degree of 'terminological inexactitude' could be demonstrated for areas other than dermatology, but the above will suffice to indicate the difficulties which get in the way of literature compilation and communication in just this one field.

Overall clinical features of patients with delusional disorder, somatic subtype

The primary feature is a persistent delusional system of a hypochondriacal or somatic nature, occurring in a setting of clear consciousness and not due to an underlying physical illness or to a psychiatric disorder other than delusional disorder. The onset may be gradual or sudden, and over a period of time the severity of the delusion may fluctuate, but in most cases the illness is unremitting and probably permanent. The patient is convinced of the physical nature of his complaint and presents it with utter conviction. He may go to extraordinary lengths to seek treatment, but the treatment is what he, rather than a physician, deems appropriate. On a cross-sectional basis, his requests may seem not unreasonable but over the long haul his preoccupation with his condition and the demands for inappropriate treatments can be seen as inappropriate and even bizarre. Lack of therapeutic success does not deter him but only seems to spur him on to obtain more and more opinions and interventions.

Perhaps half of the patients report that they 'see', 'feel' or 'smell' abnormalities and cannot be shaken from their descriptions. In some cases they may be hallucinated but more often they appear to suffer from delusional misperceptions.

Over-alerting and high anxiety seem to be almost constant features of these patients, especially when in their delusional mode (see p.50). When discussing other topics they may calm down considerably but the switch to the hyper-alert state on mention of the delusion is quite striking. Despite a rather haughty and demanding air, many will eventually admit to feelings of shame, dejection and even despair over their unremitting symptoms. Suicidal thoughts are not that uncommon and delusional disorder patients probably have a significant level of suicidal behaviour and actual suicide (Munro, 1982). Sleep deprivation seems rather frequent, partly due to agitation and partly due to night activities, such as constant cleaning to get rid of parasites. (One patient said, not without rueful humour, 'You would know my flat at night if you passed it. It's the one with the lights on and all its windows steamed up because I wash my bedclothes at least three times a night!')

Delusional disorder is synonymous with paranoia and the latter is usually associated in our minds with persecutory ideas and 'paranoid' irritability and anger. Certainly these do occur in the somatic subtype but one is often surprised to find that patients may be very wary of being sent to a psychiatrist but show no evidence of psychotic suspiciousness. They are difficult to engage therapeutically and yet, once their confidence has been gained, will often become quite willing to enter into a dialogue while remaining sceptical about the usefulness of psychiatric help in their case. Let us consider here a fairly typical case, one with a dysmorphic delusion.

Case No. 2 Delusional disorder, somatic subtype, with dysmorphic delusion

A man of 26 was referred for a psychiatric opinion. He had been attending a plastic surgery outpatient clinic and had become enraged because the surgeon had refused to operate on his face. He attacked the surgeon and two of the clinic nurses, fortunately doing no serious harm. He was arrested, but let out on bail, and his family physician requested an urgent psychiatric appointment.

The patient was remorseful about his behaviour but said he had been pinning his hopes on an operation for the previous three years and could not contain his frustration when told that he could not have it. He had a fairly obvious lower motor neuron palsy of the left seventh cranial nerve and he was convinced that people were laughing at him and talking about him because of this. He was utterly preoccupied with this belief and was convinced that only a cosmetic operation would change the situation, and would not accept the opinion of several surgeons that intervention might make the situation worse.

As a young adult he severely abused alcohol and several drugs, mainly amphetamines and cannabis. When intoxicated he could be violent and, at the age of 22, he got into a knife fight. He was stabbed in the left side of the face and was knocked unconscious, but made a good recovery. The only sequela was the deformity of the left facial region. For about a year after the fight, he had led a relatively quiet life and did not appear to have any undue concerns. Then he started to feel that people were staring at him and mocking him, and he could not rid himself of this conviction. He began to drink intermittently but heavily again, and his sense of tension only became worse. No one had suggested that surgery would be beneficial and his belief that an operation would magically cure him seemed to develop alongside his delusions of reference.

He was very disparaging about the possibility of receiving worthwhile help from psychiatry, but after a long discussion he agreed that he would tentatively try a course of neuroleptics. This was started at a low dose to avoid side effects, but for the first week he experienced some dystonia of the facial and laryngeal muscles and had to be encouraged to continue. An antiparkinsonian drug quickly improved the dystonia and after two weeks of treatment his mood began to improve rapidly, his preoccupation disappeared and he stopped hiding his face. He began to socialise again and reported that he had much less need for alcohol.

At one-year follow-up his improvement was maintained, he did not worry about his appearance and he had no desire for surgery. He was very willingly continuing to take his psychotropic medication.

Other features associated with delusional disorder, somatic subtype

In the author's own series of patients with delusional disorder, somatic subtype, an interesting set of associated features was found: demographic, behavioural and illness-related. The following comments are largely derived from personal experience (Munro, 1982).

Demographic factors

In previous publications, various estimates of frequency of the sexes were made, usually saying that women predominated over men. In this writer's series, the sexes were approximately equal but, on average, the men were considerably younger than the women, although the age ranges overlapped. As a group, the young men appeared socially unsuccessful, with unemployment problems and personality factors seeming to be almost as important as the delusional illness.

Delusional disorder patients in general appear to show an excess tendency towards celibacy and separation or divorce, and their reproductive rate is lower than normal, even in those who have been married.

It might be argued that these features are due to the adverse effects of the illness itself, but it was found that, except for approximately 20 per cent of individuals whose illness began particularly early, the onset of symptoms was late enough (average 33.8 years in males and 46.4 years in females) not to interfere seriously with upward social mobility. On the other hand, premorbid personality factors may be very important and this influence will shortly be mentioned.

Behavioural factors

Both males and females with delusional disorder have a strong tendency to regard themselves as markedly introvert, but the men especially see this as a disadvantage, leading to impaired social relationships and work performance. In these males, poor social skills probably prevented them seeking out sexual partners or, if they did form relationships, ensured that these did not succeed in a considerable proportion of cases. In the women, the process seemed a more passive one, and apparently caused less distress. However, in both sexes, there appeared to be a marked degree of social isolation even before the onset of the delusional illness, and this isolation became worse as the illness progressed. This scenario is one in which delusions, once established, tend to flourish because of a relative lack of reality input.

Once the illness is established, patients with delusional disorder, somatic subtype, show certain very characteristic behaviours. They attend multiple physicians and undergo numerous physical investigations and treatments. A sizeable minority complains bitterly about the inadequate medical treatment they have received, sometimes not without cause since the physicians often do not understand the patient's true condition and prescribe totally inappropriate treatments. Because this type of individual is so importunate and, at least in the short term, highly persuasive, many doctors respond with remarkable naîvete to their demands, then become angry and rejecting when they decide that the patient is somehow manipulating or malingering. As mentioned elsewhere, some patients initiate 'treatments' of their own, sometimes of an alarming nature.

Most of the patients experience enormous turmoil in their personal lives as a result of their extremely prolonged illness, and the families are often dragged into this. Unfortunately, the more unhappy and delusional the patient becomes, the more frantically he or she seeks the wrong kind of help and, even when in utter despair, they will usually reject contemptuously any suggestion of psychiatric help.

Illness factors

In the author's series, men were much more likely than women to have abused alcohol or other addictive substances (often in the past rather than in the present), and were also more likely to have sustained significant head injury at some time in their lives. This seemed a possible reason why the illness appears to develop earlier on average in men since their brains may well have been made more vulnerable by alcohol, drugs or injury, or a combination of more than one of these. Interestingly, but anecdotally, it seems from personally reviewed cases that women who have abused drugs or alcohol in earlier life are also more likely to develop a delusional disorder at a younger age than usual.

A background history of psychiatric disorder prior to the onset of the delusional disorder was present in one-third of these cases, but there was no previous history of psychotic illness and many of the contacts with psychiatry appeared to be related to personality difficulties or, in a few cases, to alcohol-related problems. Dejection and even depression occur in some patients after the onset of delusional disorder and probably as a reaction to this, suicidal thinking and even suicidal behaviour occur in a sizeable minority. Following treatment, as noted in Chapter 16, another sizeable minority may develop post-psychotic depression.

The family history pattern is interesting: 30 per cent of the author's patients said that there was psychiatric illness in close relatives, usually their parents or siblings, but details are scanty. The impression was that paranoid or schizophrenic illnesses are uncommon in the families, and there is evidence from elsewhere that neither schizophrenic nor mood disorders appear in excess in the families of delusional disorder patients (Watt, Hall and Olley, 1980; Kendler and Gruenberg, 1982).

The high frequency of alcohol and substance abuse and of head injury in the males is interesting, since paranoid illnesses have been described as a long-term consequence of these (Munro, 1982). One wonders whether patients whose brains undergo relatively subtle damage, or whose neurotransmitters are significantly deranged, become excessively prone to delusional disorder as an outcome. In the case of the female patients, it appears that the majority of them have to wait until changes in the ageing brain begin to produce similar effects.

Specific delusional contents of the somatic subtype

In the category of patients which is being discussed, the great majority fell into three groups with regard to the content of their delusional system, and other authors have noted that these seem to be universally the most common. They are:

(1) Delusions regarding the skin, especially infestation delusions.
(2) Delusions of ugliness or misshapenness (dysmorphic delusions).
(3) Delusions concerning body odour or halitosis.
(4) Other delusional contents which have been reported include having an abnormal dental condition (Scott and Humphreys, 1987), spreading disease (Munro, 1982), being infected with venereal disease, nowadays especially AIDS (Mahorney and Cavenar, 1988), or reporting persistent pain of bizarre nature or distribution (Malinow and Grace, 1984), etc.

Delusional disorder of all the subtypes, contrary to tradition (which says this is an illness of middle and old age), can begin at any age from adolescence onwards. There seems to be an equal chance of the onset being sudden or insidious and often the patient attributes the onset to some incident, but the veracity of this is usually difficult to check. As mentioned before, without treatment the condition usually seems to be chronic.

The frequency of the illness (delusional disorder of all types or specifically of the somatic subtype) is totally unknown, but the often repeated statement that it is rare is untrue, although it is certainly true that only a tiny minority ever reaches a psychiatrist.

We shall now look at each of the major variations on the theme of delusional disorder, somatic subtype.

Dermatological presentations

In a valuable overview of the field of psychodermatology, van Moffaert (1992) reminds us of the close interrelationships between skin and psyche. They have a shared embryological origin and also many functional links. Skin is an important tactile organ responding constantly to the external environment but also to internal emotional stimuli. It plays an essential part in tactile communication and thus in sexual relationships. Also, the skin can respond to psychological stress factors with blushing and itch and, because it is so accessible, this enables the patient to scratch or excoriate, thereby creating lesions or worsening those already there.

Dermatologists have long been aware of the clinical aspects of skin–mind interaction and there is a considerable literature on this, often ignored by psychiatrists, which will shortly be mentioned.

In this section, the dermatological presentations of delusional disorder will be considered. These can manifest in a number of different ways as follows (Lyell, 1983; Reilly and Batchelor, 1986; Wykoff, 1987; de Leon, Antelo and Simpson, 1992; Driscoll and colleagues, 1993; Baker, Cook and Winokur, 1995):

(1) Delusion of skin infestation by an insect: the patient insists that he has insects crawling over the surface of, or burrowing into, the skin. He or she may deny seeing the creatures or may describe them graphically, in which case the possibility of an associated visual hallucinatory experience must be considered. (In this author's view, such hallucinations may sometimes occur but often the description is more like a graphic ideational depiction due to the patient's extreme conviction of the presence of creatures.)

(2) A delusion of parasites burrowing under the skin. This is often attributed to worms and the rippling of small muscles below the skin's surface is sometimes interpreted as movements of the worms. Sometimes the patients believe that the worms are spread throughout the body or that they migrate from one place to another. One of this writer's patients insisted that she had worms beneath her skin which migrated each month to her breasts to mate. As evidence of the latter she said that her breasts swelled just before a menstrual period and that she could feel lumps in them. (She had chronic mastitis and probably did have lumps there, but denied feeling them at other times of the month.)

(3) Delusions of foreign bodies under the skin, sometimes described as parasites' eggs, or seed-like objects, or occasionally mineral inclusions. In some patients this is associated with an irresistible desire to pick and quite deep lesions may result. Another patient of the author's experience was covered in sores all over her body except between her shoulder blades, the only place she could not reach. She described how she would dig down with her nails until she finally found the 'worm' – a tiny, string-like creature – which may, in fact, have been a small piece of peripheral nerve tissue! People like this are often labelled as having 'neurotic excoriations' or 'factitious disorder' and are regarded as inducing their lesions deliberately. Treatment on the basis of such pseudo-diagnosis is a total failure.

(4) Less commonly, a patient will complain of giving off a foul odour, sometimes attributed to excessive sweating or to a belief that the sweat is somehow abnormal. (The picture is complicated if the person does indeed have hyperhidrosis.) This condition is further described on pp.91–94.

(5) Least common of all in psychiatric practice is chronic cutaneous dysaesthesia (Koblenzer and Bostrom, 1994), which is associated with abnormal skin sensations and sometimes glossodynia or vulvodynia. Occasionally, this is apparently due to a delusional disorder.

It should be noted that all of the above presentations may occur in a variety of psychiatric disorders, psychotic and nonpsychotic. Therefore, when one of the presenting symptoms is detected, a careful differential diagnostic process (see Chapter 2) must be undertaken to ensure that one is actually dealing with delusional disorder *per se*.

How the patient presents in delusional infestation

Very many of the patients who have delusions relating to the skin have already attended multiple dermatologists. Their story is that they contracted an infestation, sometimes insidiously but often on a specific occasion which they can describe with great precision. (One of the writer's patients *knew* that she had been infested from a towel in a motel where she and her husband had stayed overnight five years previously and which she was convinced had been unclean.) It is not inconceivable that some patients did initially have a real infestation, or a series of mosquito bites or a skin lesion interpreted as an insect bite, but they may well be in the minority.

By the time of referral to a psychiatrist, many of the patients are convinced that the physicians they have seen are incompetent since their treatments have been unavailing. They are frequently angry and distressed and are usually totally disbelieving about any help a psychiatrist may be able to give. Quite a large number, in fact, simply refuse to see the psychiatrist at all.

As with all paranoid patients, the manner is often demanding, strident and rather arrogant. The history always returns to the physical symptoms and the individual's well-rehearsed explanation of them. 'Proof' is not uncommonly presented, with an insistence on displaying skin lesions, deformed nails, bald patches, etc., and a very typical behaviour is production of what the patient insists is insect 'corpses' or 'ova', and which is usually dried lint, mucus or skin scrapings. This is known as the 'matchbox sign' (*Lancet*, 1983) in Great Britain, or the 'pill-bottle sign' in North America, as the individual usually carries his 'evidence' with him in these containers.

The patients will tell the psychiatrist at great length about their repeated attempts to disinfest themselves and their surroundings, on their own initiative or by calling in public health authorities or disinfestation experts. Sometimes belongings, furniture and even pets are disposed of in the process. Stripping themselves and their bed and washing themselves and their clothes umpteen times a day is common. Dissatisfied with their treatment, some patients start using their own treatment methods, which may become both bizarre and dangerous, and one has seen individuals who have been applying boiling hot compresses or corrosive substances to their skin to root out the insects. Despite the lack of success, patients who did these dangerous things seemed reluctant to give them up.

Some sufferers are desperately ashamed of having parasites. Others are terrified that they will pass them on to others. The result in both cases is increasing social isolation. As in other forms of delusional disorder, *folie à deux* (shared psychotic disorder, DSMIV; induced delusional disorder, ICD10) occurs in a proportion of cases and then another person, usually a close relative, will spuriously corroborate the patient's story and may even claim to be infested too.

Despite their unassailable belief, the distress they suffer and the enormous amount of time and energy they spend on their disorder and attempts for cure, a considerable number of delusional disorder patients continue to utilize the normal part of their personality to lead some kind of ongoing life. In some cases, other people do not suspect their problem or the anguish they go through. However, since the illness tends to be chronic and, unless the appropriate treatment is given, unrelenting, the individual begins sooner or later to feel despair and may even become clinically depressed. After many years of illness there may be an almost resigned attitude and the patient continues to go through the motions of demanding help, but with less vehemence. This does not always occur and one meets with patients with a 10- or 15-year history of parasitosis still demanding to see the newest dermatologist in town and refusing to accept any psychiatric help.

Other dermatological presentations related to delusional disorder

These presentations, mainly trichotillomania, onychotillomania (Hamann, 1982; Stein and Hollander, 1992), and chronic cutaneous dysaesthesia, appear to be much less common than delusional infestation and, in the great majority of cases, are more likely to be related to conditions such as personality disorder, anxiety disorder or obsessive–compulsive disorder. However, in a small proportion of cases the aetiology is actually that of a delusional disorder with its characteristic features, although there may be some difficulty in confirming this in a patient who refuses to accept a psychological explanation.

Some cases of hair plucking or nail removal are symptomatic of infestation delusions, the individual removing hair or nails as the result of a compulsive gouging process. One of the writer's patients, an elderly woman, believed delusionally that she had bugs burrowing under her nails and had picked the nails down to the nail beds to expose them. She appeared unaware of what she was doing: during interview she incessantly picked but, when asked, denied that she was doing any damage to her nails which she insisted had been destroyed by the insects.

In these cases, the management and treatment approach is as with the infestation delusions and these will be discussed more generally later.

Case No 3   Delusional disorder, somatic subtype, with delusions of infestation

A woman in her late 40s reported that, 12 years earlier, she had been undergoing divorce and was under great stress at that time. She developed a skin itch which fairly rapidly spread all over her body, and after a time she became convinced that she had insects burrowing under her skin. She never saw these creatures, but could feel them and experienced pain from their bites. Her preoccupation with the 'infestation' became almost total and she visited many dermatologists without obtaining any relief from their treatments. (Her family physician reported that none of the dermatologists found any evidence of infestation.) She gave up work, withdrew from social activities, and slept poorly. She washed herself incessantly, even getting up at night several times to shower, and also washed her clothes several times a day. She had used various applications on her skin, including bleach, which had caused painful lesions. At one time she used to gouge out the 'lumps' but now prevented herself from doing this.

There was a lifelong psychiatric history. She had a severely unstable and unhappy childhood and had always been 'highly strung'. She overdosed at the age of 10, and at about the same time she suffered a skull fracture in a fall. A sister committed suicide and she herself had overdosed twice in the 10 years prior to the present time. During the 12 years that she had suffered from her symptoms she had been treated with tricyclics, phenothiazines and benztropines, without effect.

At interview she was distraught and preoccupied with her complaint, which she held to with total conviction. However, when she calmed down somewhat, she could talk relatively calmly about other matters and there was no evidence of widespread delusions or of thought disorder. She was reluctant to accept help from a psychiatrist but was eventually persuaded to take a neuroleptic. After a week she was much less distressed and after two weeks the 'biting' was considerably diminished. Sleep began to improve, and after five weeks of treatment she complained of only mild residual itching. She said the insects had gone, but still fully believed that they had been there.

Follow-up after six months revealed that she had obtained permanent work and had resumed a social life. She said that she felt emotionally more stable than she had done for years. Despite her lack of insight she was very prepared to continue taking the neuroleptic and she was referred back to her family doctor for prolonged follow-up.

Delusional disorder, somatic subtype, with a dysmorphic delusion

Earlier in this chapter a sequence was described in which some individuals are seen to progress from normal to abnormal health concern, to persistent somatization or even to psychiatric illness with somatization features. Delusional disorder, somatic subtype, may be one of these illnesses, and one of its presentations is with a delusion of dysmorphic content, which may be seen as one type of abnormality of the body image or schema. In Case No. 2 a typical example of this is described (see p.81).

Once again, nomenclature is a stumbling block and, in particular, the frequent use of the term dysmorphophobia is a potent cause of confusion. The term is an old one (Morselli, 1886) and literally means a fear of being misshapen. Unfortunately, over the years its usage became very loose and the present author and a colleague (Munro and Stewart, 1991) were able to identify six separate meanings attributed to it at various times. Many authors who use it fail to define their understanding of it and it is impossible to be certain of the nature of the cases they describe; in many instances their series almost certainly contain a mixture of diagnoses, including both delusional and nondelusional patients. Munro and Stewart (1991) proposed that we use the descriptive word 'dysmorphic' to indicate a patient's belief of being abnormal in shape or appearance: however, it would be necessary to qualify this as a symptom, a complaint or a delusion and also to state which specific syndrome was being alluded to. Schachter (1971) presaged this viewpoint to some extent when he described 'dysmorphia' and divided cases into neurotic and psychotic subgroups, and Thomas (1990, 1995) makes a clear distinction between delusional disorder of the somatic subtype and nonpsychotic types of 'dysmorphophobia'. However, some authors cling to the belief that dysmorphophobia is a diagnosis in itself and covers all types of dysmorphic conviction (de Leon, Bott and Simpson, 1989). As a variation on this theme, Phillips (1991) and Phillips and colleagues (1993) suggest the possibility that body dysmorphic disorder (a nondelusional illness) may have a psychotic subtype and that this is possibly on a continuum with delusional disorder with dysmorphic beliefs. The present author believes that this suggestion unnecessarily blurs diagnostic boundaries between two very distinct illnesses, and the topic will be considered again in Chapter 12.

As in all subtypes of delusional disorder, that with a dysmorphic delusion will present with a stable, encapsulated delusional system in the setting of a relatively normal personality. The dysmorphic delusion will vary according to the individual patient and examples include a conviction of personal ugliness, an insistence on misshapenness or a belief that a body part is overprominent or unduly small, all remaining unshaken by evidence to the contrary. (A subtype of delusion regarding body size is that occasionally found in association with severe anorexia or bulimia (see Chapter 15)). Any part of the body may be picked out for concern (Pruzinsky, 1988).

The diagnosis of dysmorphic delusion is often far from easy. As Snaith (1992) points out, there are social influences on our perception of body shape and body size and these have become particularly strong in recent years, with undue emphasis on slenderness, especially in young women. Dissatisfaction with body shape can begin even in children (Salmons and colleagues, 1988), and Braddock (1982) describes how difficult diagnosis can be in a 'dysmorphophobic' adolescent, when sociopsychological and psychopathological influences may be inextricably intertwined.

Highly demanding patients with dysmorphic convictions often find their way to plastic or cosmetic surgeons, and there is a literature related to these specialties which is relevant to delusional disorder. Unfortunately, in most cases the surgeon is apt to underestimate the influence of psychological factors in complaining characteristics and may be only too ready to operate, even when the patient's motivations are highly suspect (Hawes and Bible, 1990). There is everything to be said for collaboration between surgeons and mental health specialists in screening prospective patients for plastic surgery – especially those whose appearance does not appear to justify their complaint – and in a few centres this is accepted (Pruzinsky, 1988). However, psychiatrists are mostly still uninvolved in this area of medical practice and have no idea of the extent of the problem or the potentially calamitous outcome of performing inappropriate surgery on deluded patients (Pruzinsky and Edgerton, 1990). This is commended as a potentially important area for inter-specialty co-operation.

Delusional disorder, somatic subtype, with a delusion of smell

Pryse-Phillips, a neurologist, produced a paper in 1971 on the 'olfactory reference syndrome', a disorder which was, he said, characterized by *hallucinations* of smell. He studied 99 cases of his own and cited another 38 individuals, all with this type of hallucination. He claimed that the patients could be divided into four groups, those with depressive illness, those with schizophrenia, a group with temporal lobe epilepsy and, finally, patients with the 'olfactory reference syndrome' who somewhat resembled depressives. His series is probably the most extensive in the literature so far, and has been widely quoted, but his olfactory reference syndrome does not fit comfortably into any current psychiatric diagnostic system.

Other authors, for example Bishop (1980) and Davidson and Mukherjee (1982), use the term 'olfactory reference syndrome' as though it were the standard term for an illness whose principal feature was a *delusion* of smell, and describe in one instance a case of apparent delusional disorder and in another a case of bipolar mood disorder with this symptom.

Neurologists are familiar with hallucinations related to temporal lobe epilepsy, in which patients report the sensation of a variety of odours, mainly unpleasant. Usually this is not referred to the self and the patient does not normally report that he is giving off the smell. In psychiatric disorders in which the patient insistently reports a smell, it may not be clear whether this is a hallucination or (as is more often likely) a delusion. These patients may say that the smell emanates from them and is evident to others. If they can describe the nature of the smell closely, it may be regarded as a hallucination as well as a delusion. On the other hand, many patients say that they know they give off an unpleasant smell because other people look disgusted and move away from them, but the smell is not apparent to themselves: in this instance, they are suffering from a delusion. The smell may be attributed to abnormal sweat, to flatus leaking from the bowel or to severe halitosis (Goldberg, Buongiorno and Henkin, 1985; Iwu and Akpata, 1989).

Nomenclature is once again messy. As well as olfactory reference syndrome there are references to delusions of bromosis (from the Greek word 'to stink': bromine is the 'stinking element'), delusions of smell, olfactory delusional syndrome, delusional halitosis, hallucinatory halitosis and imaginary halitosis. In their article on delusional halitosis, Iwu and Akpata (1989) describe it as a variation of olfactory reference syndrome and give the following characteristics for their patients:

Onset is relatively early (mean 25 years).
There is an excess of males and an excess of the unmarried.
None of the patients had had prior psychiatric treatment.
There is an incessant search for medical treatment.

The personality remains integrated and social life is maintained. The individual's life is dominated by the belief. Some patients have secondary depression.

The diagnoses of the cases in this article are unclear but the description given above might apply equally to a delusional disorder group or to body dysmorphic disorder (see Chapter 12). In the small literature on delusions of smell, a number of psychiatric disorders is mentioned, including unipolar and bipolar mood disorder (including psychotic depression), schizophrenia (including paranoid schizophrenia), delusional disorder and atypical paranoid disorder.

There are undoubtedly some cases of smell delusion (with or without associated hallucination) which can be diagnosed as delusional disorder, somatic subtype, but references to these are few. There is an occasional reference to the efficacy of pimozide in such cases (Littler, 1986; Malasi and colleagues, 1990; Ulzen, 1993). Otherwise, the treatment is presumably that of whatever other psychiatric disorder underlies the symptom.

When we are discussing a delusional disorder with a delusion of smell, the designation of the condition should be, 'delusional disorder, somatic subtype, characterized by a delusion of smell'.

Case No. 4   Delusional disorder, somatic subtype, with a delusion of smell

A woman aged 63 began to attend her family physician much more frequently than usual with a variety of rather vague physical complaints. On one of her visits, clearly distressed and embarrassed, she broke down and told him that she had a severe bowel problem which caused her to pass evil-smelling flatus all the time. A devout churchgoer, she was no longer able to attend church because people sitting near her would wrinkle their noses and move away from her. This had gone on for about two months and she finally gave up attending because she was sure she heard an elder use her name and say to another, 'don't take her collection, she smells badly'.

She had given up all her social activities and would not even visit her married children because she believed that they, and her grandchildren, were backing away from her and were pulling faces in her presence. The only person she could tolerate being near her was her husband because he 'had chronic sinusitis and no sense of smell'.

The family doctor could find no physical abnormality but ordered some investigations and obtained a consultation from a gastroenterologist who told the patient her bowel was perfectly normal. This distressed her because she 'knew' the problem was continuing unabated. She felt enormous shame, remained reclusive and had thoughts of suicide because life was not worth living.

She was given antianxiety and antidepressant medications with no avail and was then referred to a psychiatrist for assessment. He changed her to another antidepressant which was equally unhelpful. There then followed a period of several months during which the patient became more and more distraught and finally took an overdose of her antidepressant. After resuscitation in hospital she was admitted to an inpatient psychiatric unit where a more extensive history was obtained. The diagnosis was changed to delusional disorder, somatic subtype, and a suitable neuroleptic was instituted. The patient was very compliant and during a two-week hospital stay her conviction about the smell diminished considerably. Following discharge she conscientiously took her medication, said the smell had vanished and was able gradually to return to her social activities. A year later her family physician stopped her neuroleptic because she appeared so well. Within three weeks her 'bad smell' began to reappear and she demanded that her neuroleptic be reinstated. She remains well at this time.

Delusional disorder, somatic subtype, with facial and dental symptoms

Marbach (1978) described the so-called 'phantom bite syndrome' with which some dentists are familiar. Here, the patient insists against evidence that his dental bite is abnormal and repeatedly demands corrective treatment, often from many dentists in succession. One tooth after another will be built up or ground down, but the result is never satisfactory and the patient's demands only become more insistent.

In a similar vein, Malinow and Grace (1984) report on facial pain and monodelusional illness in two patients in which no satisfactory focus for the pain could ever be found. The patients both insisted on mass extractions of teeth, but never with any beneficial result. The authors suggest that this is a not uncommon problem in dental practice, and Marbach and colleagues, (1983) note that such patients are a 'source of great frustration, financial loss and potential litigation'. Elsewhere, Marbach (1985) suggests that dentists should learn to recognize monodelusional patients, should avoid operating on them if at all possible, and should consider treatment with pimozide or haloperidol in the unlikely event that the patient will accept it.

Scott and Humphreys (1987) also describe the phantom bite syndrome and, in addition, patients with dysmorphic beliefs that the jaw is deformed and that this is noticeable to other people, despite evidence to the contrary. As is typical in such cases, they go to many different specialists demanding surgical treatment. These authors also suggest pimozide as the treatment of choice.

Finally, and somewhat of an oddity even in this field of strange complaints, Mack (1985) reports on an elderly man with atherosclerotic brain disorder and a monodelusional belief that a thick growth of hair kept recurring on his dentures! There was clearly a *folie à deux* situation here, as his wife solemnly confirmed his complaint. The delusion disappeared completely after eight weeks' treatment with pimozide. Mack, perhaps rather tongue in cheek, comments that this may be the first reported case in which the delusion had become fixed on a prosthesis rather than on a natural part of the body.

The designation of cases of this general type is 'delusional disorder, somatic subtype, characterized by a delusion of dental abnormality/dental pain'.

Case No. 5   Delusional disorder, somatic subtype, with complaint of dental malocclusion

A colleague in dental surgery gave an account of two male patients whom he had treated at the same time, both of whom caused him considerable exasperation and concern. Each man complained of malocclusion problems which did not resolve with repeated dental interventions.

The first patient, a man of 52, had apparently had no difficulty with his teeth until a few months before, then started to feel that his bite had become uncomfortable to him. He visited his dentist who replaced a couple of fillings and made an adjustment to a partial dental plate. This produced no improvement and the patient returned on an increasingly frequent basis, complaining of discomfort when chewing, although otherwise behaving quite reasonably. After several attempts to correct the bite, the dentist decided that the complaint was 'neurotic' and referred the man to his family physician.

The second patient was aged 35 and had recently moved from a distant city and presented to the dentist with a very insistent demand that he make a new upper denture for him since the present one did not fit. Examination showed no obvious abnormality but when the dentist offered to repair the denture the patient showed anger and said he needed a totally new one. Somewhat reluctantly it was agreed that another denture would be made: during the next week the patient telephoned several times every day, demanding to know why it was not yet ready. When he came for a fitting he was irritable and refused to accept the new prosthesis, saying it was extremely painful. For the next several weeks there were numerous consultations, adjustments of the denture and escalating recriminations by the patient who eventually accused the dentist of incompetence and stormed out. For several weeks he went on telephoning the dentist, making various insulting remarks, then contact ceased.

The first patient's general practitioner contacted the dentist to say that physical examination had revealed slight spasticity of the orofacial muscles and fibrillation of the tongue. He had made a provisional diagnosis of amyotrophic lateral sclerosis and referred the man to a neurologist for investigation. It seemed that the 'dental' discomfort was a misinterpretation by the patient of the early motor symptoms of his neurological disorder. He died of this disorder about nine months later.

When he submitted his insurance claim for the second patient, the dentist was visited by a claims investigator from the company who said that the man had attended numerous dentists in several cities over the previous five years and had had more than a hundred interventions, all for the complaint of malocclusion. He apparently went through the same process with each practitioner, demanding treatments and eventually rejecting each with scurrilous accusations. Attempts by the company to contact the man always proved unavailing because of his extreme mobility. The dentist in the present account never heard from him again.

Despite the apparent similarity of their complaints, these two patients had entirely different disorders. Patient number one was in the early states of a potentially fatal nervous system disease. It seems probable that the other man suffered from delusional disorder, somatic subtype, with a delusion of dental malocclusion – the condition sometimes referred to as the 'phantom bite syndrome' (Marbach, 1978).

Delusional disorder, somatic subtype, in relation to anorexia nervosa and bulimia nervosa (Birtchnell, Lacey and Harte, 1985; Cooper and Taylor, 1988)

The great majority of cases of anorexia nervosa are not associated with delusions, but elsewhere (Chapter 12) it is suggested that a small number of patients who apparently have anorexia nervosa may actually have a mono-delusional illness centring around appearance, weight and eating. The author's personal views on this have been suggested by a very small number of cases in which undoubtedly delusional individuals developed very strange beliefs on food and adopted bizarre diets.

Plantey (1977) reports a dramatic response to pimozide in a youth of 17 with anorexia nervosa and he quotes Barry and Klawans (1976) who propose an aetiological theory for the illness based on dopaminergic receptor activity and suggesting treatment with pimozide. Unfortunately, it does not seem as though there has been any systematic follow-up of these authors' theories.

Anorexic and bulimic cases are very common and this particular variation may be rare, but it is still important to identify such patients since their treatment would be very different from the conventional approach to eating disorders. The designation would be 'delusional disorder, somatic subtype, with eating disorder features'.

A case of delusional anorexia is described in Chapter 12.

Delusional disorder, somatic subtype, with a delusion of sexually transmitted disease

In 1978, Bhanji and Mahony reported that a number of patients attending a venereal disease clinic, but who had no evidence of physical disorder, were deluded and responded to pimozide.

Schizophrenics and, even more so, psychotically depressed individuals, not infrequently believe quite falsely that they have contracted a sexually transmitted disease. Traditionally the favourite was syphilis but in recent years the preoccupation with AIDS has deposed that disorder.

Frost (1985), in a study of 100 consecutive patients referred from a venereology clinic for psychiatric assessment, found that many were very anxious or angry but had no definable psychiatric illness. Alroe (1988) described a case of AIDS 'paranoia' which was actually a mixture of phobic and depressive symptoms, but Rundell, Wise and Ursano (1986) seem to be describing delusional disorder in at least one case with AIDS delusions, although they also describe cases with depressive illness and

adjustment disorder. Other authors usually report cases which are predominantly mood disorders (including mania), schizophrenia and
schizoaffective disorder (Lawlor and Stewart, 1987; Mahorney and
Cavenar, 1988; Seymour, 1989).

An interesting variant is where the patient does indeed have AIDS and
develops a delusional disorder, perhaps as a result of organic brain
changes. Holmes (1989) reports on an individual who was HIV-positive
and who exhibited infestation delusions which responded well to pimozide.
Reilly and Batchelor (1991) discuss the possibility that infestation delusions in AIDS might arise from paraesthesiae caused by the effects of the
latter.

If a case of this type is recognized, the diagnosis is 'delusional disorder,
somatic subtype, with delusions of sexually transmitted disease (AIDS/
syphilis/other)'.

**Case No. 6   Delusional disorder, somatic subtype, with a delusion of
sexually transmitted disease (AIDS)**

A young man of 24 presented himself at the assessment service of a
department of psychiatry in a state of great distress. He said that he
had had sexual relations with a prostitute three months before and
was now convinced he had AIDS. He had been to a venereal diseases
clinic soon after the sexual contact, where he was examined and
serologically tested; he was told he had no evidence of any sexually
transmitted disease but was advised to return at regular intervals for
serial testing. Several weeks later he started to attend the clinic daily,
demanding repeat investigations, and eventually was virtually excluded, with a warning that police would be called if he continued to
harass staff.

His anxiety became intolerable and did not respond to a ben-
zodiazepine prescribed by his family physician. He then came to the
psychiatric service where, at first, he was regarded as a highly obsessional individual with severe anxiety and was prescribed a serotonergic antidepressant. Three days later he took a severe overdose of this
and was admitted in coma to a medical unit where he was resus-
citated. He was then transferred to a psychiatric inpatient unit.
There, following several days of observation, it became gradually
clear that his belief in venereal infection was delusional in intensity.

He talked incessantly about his concern, could not be dissuaded by argument or by evidence of further normal serological tests. When talking about his hypochondriacal delusion his manner was extremely tense and he was physically restless. When he could be persuaded to discuss other topics, he was much less intense and he made good sense. He had no insight into the unreasonableness of his belief. A diagnosis of delusional disorder was made.

With much persuasion he eventually agreed to take a neuroleptic drug. His compliance was uncertain, but over a period of about a week he seemed to relax a little, socialise moderately with other patients and appear a little less preoccupied. It was learned only later that at this time he told another patient that, despite some lessening of anxiety, he could not tolerate the idea of having a potentially fatal illness. In repeated clinical interviews he did not show any evidence of clinical depression or make further suicidal threats.

One day, despite close observation, he went missing from the inpatient unit and his body was discovered by the police several hours later on wasteground close to the hospital. He had stabbed himself through the heart. He left no suicide note.

Conclusion

We have illustrated some (not necessarily all) of the more important themes which can characterize delusional disorder of the somatic subtype. Patients with this illness believe unremittingly that they have a specific physical condition and insist on attending the medical specialist who deals with that condition. In the present author's experience, dermatologists seem to be the most aware of the real nature of these cases, although their nomenclature may be uncertain. But infectious and tropical disease specialists also have an awareness of the disorder because some of their patients have delusions of infestation, and venereologists report on patients with a mistaken conviction of having a sexually transmitted disease. At one end of the bowel, dentists see patients who have delusional complaints of malocclusion or halitosis while, at the other, gastroenterologists deal with individuals who believe that their bowel gives off a foul smell. And so on.

Generally speaking, psychiatrists do not see these cases unless a specific specialist requests a consultation. If one works in a psychiatric consultation–liaison service in a large general hospital and has an interest in delusional disorder, cases of the somatic subtype will start to trickle in and, as the author can confirm from experience, it is not difficult to build up a series. It is essential that we psychiatrists should be knowledgeable about the clinical features and treatment of the illness. Successful treatment of these patients can often result in gratifying therapeutic outcomes (see Chapter 16) and can win the undying gratitude of medical colleagues who have been incessantly harassed by these unhappy, importunate and dissatisfied individuals.

References

Alexander, J. O'D. (1984). Delusion of cutaneous parasitosis In *Arthropods and Human Skin*, ed. J. O'D. Alexander. pp 391–398. Berlin: Springer-Verlag.
Alroe, C.J. (1988). AIDS paranoia. *Med. J. Aust.* **148**: 369 (letter).
Baker, P.B., Cook, B.L. and Winokur, G. (1995). Delusional infestation: the interface of delusions and hallucinations. *Psychiat. Clin. N. Am.* **18**: 345–362.
Barry, V.C. and Klawans, A.C. (1976). *J. Neurol. Transmiss.* **38**: 107 *quoted* by F. Plantey, (1977). *Lancet* **1**: 1105.
Barsky, A.J., Wyshak, G., Klerman, G.L. and Latham, K.S. (1990). The prevalence of hypochondriasis in medical outpatients. *Soc. Psychiat. Psychiat. Epidemiol.* **25**: 89–94.
Berrios, G.E. (1982). Tactile hallucinations: conceptual and historical aspects. *J. Neurol. Neurosurg. Psychiat.* **45**: 285–293.
Bhanji, S. and Mahony, J.D.H. (1978). The value of a psychiatric service within the venereal disease clinic. *Br. J. Vener. Dis.* **54**: 266–268.
Birtchnell, S.A., Lacey, J.H. and Harte, A. (1985). Body image distortion in bulimia nervosa. *Br. J. Psychiat.* **147**: 408–412.
Bishop, E.R. (1980). Monosymptomatic hypochondriasis. *Psychosomatics* **21**: 731–747.
Braddock, L.E. (1982). Dysmorphophobia in adolescence: a case report. *Br. J. Psychiat.* **140**: 199–201.
Brink, T.L., Capri, D., Deneeve, V., Janakes, C. and Oliveira, C. (1979). Hypochondriasis and paranoia. *J. Nerv. Ment. Dis.* **167**: 224–228.
Cash, T.F. and Pruzinsky, T. (eds) (1990). *Body Images: Development, Deviance and Change*. New York: Guilford Press.
Cooper, P.J. and Taylor, M.J. (1988). Body image disturbance in bulimia nervosa. *Br. J. Psychiat.* **153** (supplement 2) : 32–36.
Cumming, W.J.K. (1988). The neurobiology of the body schema. *Br. J. Psychiat.* **153** (supplement 2) : 7–11.
Davidson, M. and Mukherjee, S. (1982). Progression of olfactory reference syndrome to mania: a case report. *Am. J. Psychiat.* **139**: 1623–1624.
Dean, J.T., Nelson, E. and Moss, L. (1992). Pathologic hair-pulling: a review of the literature and case reports. *Comprehens. Psychiat.* **33**: 84–91.
Diagnostic and Statistical Manual of Mental Disorders, 3rd edn, revised (DSMIIIR) (1987). Washington, DC American Psychiatric Association.
Diagnostic and Statistical Manual of Mental Disorders, 4th edn (DSMIV) (1994). Washington: American Psychiatric Association.

Driscoll, M.S., Rothe, M.J., Grant-Kels, J.M. and Hale, M.S. (1993). Delusional parasitosis: a dermatologic, psychiatric, and pharmacologic approach. *J. Am. Acad. Dermatol.* **29**:1023–1033.

Edwards, R. (1977). Delusions of parasitosis. *Br. Med. J.* **1**: 1219.

Ekbom, K.A. (1938). Der präsenile Dermatozoenwahn. *Acta Psychiatri. Neurolog. Scand.* **13**: 227–259.

Elpern, D.J. (1988). Cocaine abuse and delusions of parasitosis. *Cutis* **52**: 273–274.

Frost, D.P. (1985). Recognition of hypochondriasis in a clinic for sexually transmitted disease. *Genitourin Med.* **61**: 133–137.

Goldberg, R.L., Buongiorno, P.A. and Henkin, R.I. (1985). Delusions of halitosis. *Psychosomatics* **26**: 325–331.

Hamann, K. (1982). Onychotillomania treated with pimozide (Orap). *Acta Dermatovener (Stockholm)* **62**: 364–366.

Hawes, M.J. and Bible, H.H. (1990). The paranoid patient: surgeon beware! *Ophthal. Plast. Reconstruct. Surg.* **6**: 225–227.

Holmes, V.F. (1989). Treatment of monosymptomatic hypochondriacal psychosis with pimozide in an AIDS patient. *Am. J. Psychiat.* **146**: 554–555 (letter).

International Statistical Classification of Diseases, 10th edn (ICD10) 1992–3 Geneva: World Health Organization.

Iwu, C.O. and Akpata, O. (1989). Delusional halitosis: review of the literature and analysis of 32 cases. *Br. Dent. J.* **167**: 294–296.

Katon, W., Lin, E., Von Korff, M., Russo, J., Lipscomb, P.and Bush, T. (1991). Somatization: a spectrum of severity. *Am. J. Psychiat.* **148**: 34–40.

Kellner, R. (1992). Diagnosis and treatments of hypochondriacal syndromes. *Psychosomatics* **33**: 278–289.

Kendler, K.S. and Gruenberg, A.M. (1982). Genetic relationship between paranoid personality disorder and the 'Schizophrenic spectrum' disorders. *Am. J. Psychiat.* **139**: 1185–1187.

Koblenzer, C.S. and Bostrom, P. (1994). Chronic cutaneous dysesthesia syndrome: a psychotic phenomenon or a depressive symptom? *J. Am. Acad. Dermatol.* **30**: 370–374.

Kraepelin, E. (1921). *Manic-Depressive Insanity and Paranoia*, transl. by R. M. Barclay (1976). New York: Arno Press.

Lancet (1983). The matchbox sign (leading article) **ii**: 261.

Lawlor, B.A. and Stewart, J.T. (1987). AIDS delusions: a symptom of our times. *Am. J. Psychiat.* **144**: 1244 (letter)

de Leon, J., Antelo, R.E. and Simpson, G. (1992). Delusion of parasitosis or chronic tactile hallucinosis: hypothesis about their brain physiopathology. *Comprehens. Psychiat.* **33**: 25–33.

de Leon, J., Bott, A. and Simpson, G.M. (1989). Dysmorphophobia: body dysmorphic disorder or delusional disorder, somatic subtype. *Comprehens. Psychiat.* **30**: 457–472.

Lipowski, Z.J. (1988). Somatization: the concept and its clinical application. *Am. J. Psychiat.* **145**: 1358–1368.

Littler, C.M. (1986). Pimozide for delusions of bromosis. *J. Am. Acad. Dermatol.* **15**: 1303–1304 (letter).

Lyell, A. (1983). Delusions of parasitosis. *Sem. Dermatol.* **2**: 189–195.

Lynch, P.J. (1993). Delusions of parasitosis. *Sem. Dermatol.* **12**: 39–45.

Mack, P.J. (1985). Hairy dentures: a monosymptomatic hypochondriacal psychosis. *Br. Dent. J.* **158**: 50–51.

Mahorney, S.L. and Cavenar, J.O. (1988). A new and timely delusion: the complaint of having AIDS. *Am. J. Psychiat.* **145**: 1130–1132.

Malasi, T.H., El-Hilu, S.R., Mirza, I.A. and El-Islam, M.F. (1990). Olfactory delusional syndrome with various aetiologies. *Br. J. Psychiat.* **156**: 256–260.

Malinow, K.L. and Grace, E.G. (1984). Facial pain and monosymptomatic hypochondriasis. *J. Oral Maxillofac. Surg.* **42**: 330–332.

Marbach, J.J. (1978). Phantom bite syndrome. *Am. J. Psychiat.* **135**: 476–478.

Marbach, J.J. (1985). Psychosocial factors for failure to adapt to dental prostheses. *Dent. Clin. N. Am.* **29**: 215–233.

Marbach, J.J., Varoscak, J.R., Blank, R.T. and Lund, P. (1983). 'Phantom bite': classification and treatment. *J. Prosthet. Dent.* **49**: 556–559.

Marschall, M.A., Dolezal, R.F. and Cohen, M. (1991). Chronic wounds and delusions of parasitosis in the drug abuser. *Plast. Reconstr. Surg.* **88**: 328–330.

Morselli, E. (1886). Sulla ismorfofobia e sulla tafefobia. *Boll. Accad. Sci. Med. (Genoa)* **6**: 100–119.

Munro, A. (1982). *Delusional Hypochondriasis.* Clarke Institute of Psychiatry Monograph Series No. 5. Toronto: Clarke Institute of Psychiatry.

Munro, A. (1988). Pinpointing the true hypochondriac patient. *Diagnosis (Can. J. Diag.)* **5**: 113–123.

Munro, A. and Stewart, M. (1991). Body dysmorphic disorder and the DSMIV: the demise of dysmorphophobia. *Can. J. Psychiat.* **36**: 91–96.

Murray, S.J., Ross, J.B. and Murray, A.H. (1987). Life-threatening dermatitis artefacta. *Cutis* **39**: 387–388.

Phillips, K.A. (1991). Body dysmorphic disorder: the distress of imagined ugliness. *Am. J. Psychiat.* **148**: 1138–1149.

Phillips, K.A., McElroy, S.L., Keck, P.E., Pope, H.G. and Hudson, J.I. (1993). Body dysmorphic disorder: 30 cases of imagined ugliness. *Am. J. Psychiat.* **150**: 302–308.

Plantey, F. (1977). Pimozide in treatment of anorexia nervosa. *Lancet* **1**: 1105 (letter).

Pruzinsky, T. (1988). Collaboration of plastic surgeon and medical psychotherapist: elective cosmetic surgery. *Med. Psychother.* **1**: 1–13.

Pruzinsky, T. (1990). Psychopathology of body experience: expanded perspectives. In *Body Images: Development, Deviance and Change*, ed. T.F. Cash and T. Pruzinsky, Chap. 8, pp 170–189. New York: Guilford Press.

Pruzinsky, T. and Cash, T.F. (1990). Integrative themes in body-image development, deviance and change. In *Body Images: Development, Deviance and Change*, ed. T.F. CASH, and T. Pruzinsky, Chap. 16, pp. 337–349. New York: Guilford Press.

Pruzinsky, T. and Edgerton, M.T. (1990). Body-image change in cosmetic plastic surgery In *Body Images: Development, Deviance and Change*, ed. T.F. Cash and T. Pruzinsky, Chap. 10, pp 217–236. New York:Guilford Press.

Pryse-Phillips, W. (1971) An olfactory reference syndrome. *Acta Psychiatr. Scand.* **47**: 484–509.

Purcell, T.B. (1991). The somatic patient. *Emerg. Med. Clin. N. Am.* **9**: 137–159.

Reilly, T.M. and Batchelor, D.H. (1986). The presentation and treatment of delusional parasitosis: a dermatological perspective. *Int. Clin. Psychopharmacol.* **1**: 340–353.

Reilly, T.M. and Batchelor, D.H. (1991). Monosymptomatic hypochondriacal psychosis and AIDS. *Am. J. Psychiat.* **148**: 815 (letter).

Rundell, J.R., Wise, M.G. and Ursano, R.J. (1986). Three cases of AIDS-related psychiatric disorders. *Am. J. Psychiat.* **143**: 777–778.

Salmons, P.H., Lewis, V.J., Rogers, P., Gatherer, A.J.H. and Booth, D.A. (1988). Body shape dissatisfaction in children. *Br. J. Psychiat.* **153** (supplement 2) : 27–31.

Schachter, M. (1971). Neuroses dysmorphophobiques (complexes de laideur et délire ou conviction délirante de dysmorphophobie). *Ann. Med. Psychologiq.* **129**: 123–145.

Scott, J. and Humphreys, M. (1987). Psychiatric aspects of dentistry I. *Br. Dent. J.* **163**: 81–87.

Seymour, J. (1989). Delusions of having AIDS. *Am. J. Psychiat.* **146**: 556 (letter).

Sifneos, P.E. (1973). The prevalence of 'alexithymic' characteristics in psychosomatic patients. *Psychother. Psychosom.* **22**: 255–262.

Skott, A. (1978). Delusions of Infestation. Reports from the Psychiatric Research Centre, St. Jörgen Hospital. Göteborg, Sweden: University of Göteborg.

Snaith, P. (1992). Body image disorders. *Psychother. Psychosom.* **58**: 119–124.

Stein, D.J. and Hollander, E. (1992). Low-dose pimozide augmentation of serotonin reuptake blockers in the treatmentof trichotillomania. *J. Clin. Psychiat.* **53**: 123–126.

Tanquary, J., Lynch, M. and Masand, P. (1992). Obsessive–compulsive disorder in relation to body dysmorphic disorder. *Am. J. Psychiat.* **149**: 1283–1284 (letter).

Thomas, C.S. (1990). Body-dysmorphic disorder. *Am. J. Psychiat.* **147**: 816–817 (letter).

Thomas, C.S. (1995). A study of facial dysmorphophobia.*Psychiatr. Bull.* **19**: 736–739.

Ulzen, T.P.M. (1993) Pimozide-responsive monosymptomatic hypochondriacal psychosis in an adolescent. *Can. J. Psychiat.* **38**: 153–154 (letter).

Van Moffaert, M. (1992). Psychodermatology: an overview. *Psychother. Psychosom.* **58**: 125–136.

Warwick, H.M., Clark, D.M., Cobb, A.M. and Salkovskis, P.M. (1996). A controlled trial of cognitive-behavioural treatment of hypochondriasis. *Br. J. Psychiat.* **169**: 189–195.

Watt, J.A.G., Hall, D.J. and Olley, P.C. (1980). Paranoid states of middle life. Familiar occurrence and relationship to schizophrenia. *Acta Psychiat. Scand.* **61**: 413–426.

Wykoff, R.F. (1987). Delusions of parasitosis: a review. *Rev. Infect. Dis.* **9**: 433–437.

4

Delusional disorder, jealousy subtype

As in all areas of the literature on delusional disorders in their various forms, there is considerable confusion when discussing jealousy and it is not always clear whether authors are describing normal or pathological jealousy or, in the latter case, which associated psychiatric illness they are considering. Jealousy can arise in a variety of contexts but in this chapter we are dealing more or less exclusively with sexual jealousy. Sexual jealousy is virtually a universal human emotion: there have been anthropological descriptions of societies in which sexual partners are exchanged apparently without distress, but this seems to be excessively rare.

Most of us fully understand that jealousy is likely to arise when a rival attempts to attract away an individual's sexual partner. Interestingly, according to Mullen and Martin (1994), men and women tend to react somewhat differently in such a situation. The jealous male is likely to be more concerned about actual loss of the partner, whereas the female is more prone to worry about the effect of infidelity on the quality of the ongoing relationship. Both sexes seem equally prone to experience jealousy, however differently they express it.

There is reasonable consensus that jealousy can occur at three levels of significance. First, there is normal jealousy which can vary from mild discomfiture to savage rage, but is comprehensible in the light of the individual's situation or, at least, his understanding of it (e.g. it is possible for normal jealousy to be due to a misapprehension and the other person can be totally innocent) (Mathes, Adams and Davies, 1985). The expression of jealousy is related considerably to temperamental factors and may not always reflect accurately the individual's underlying mental state, some people readily making accusations and others habitually bottling up their feelings.

Secondly, there is so-called 'neurotic' jealousy in which the mood and its means of expression are relatively normal but, due to nonpsychotic psychiatric illness or to personality disorder, it is excessive in degree and in the readiness with which it is evoked. Here, the jealous belief is an overvalued idea but nonetheless can show considerable irrationality and recidivism, as well as excessive vehemence and even violence at times (Seeman, 1979).

Finally, there is psychotic jealousy which is characterized by delusions of jealousy which cannot be shaken by contrary argument or evidence. This has been described as occurring in association with severe mood disorder (Bishay, Petersen and Tarrier, 1989), schizophrenia or organic brain disorder (Soyka, Naber and Völcker, 1991), alcoholism (Alarcon 1980; Michael and colleagues, 1995), and paranoid or delusional disorder (Shepherd, 1961; Alarcon, 1980; Munro, 1989; Soyka, 1992). It is this last form which will be considered in particular detail in the present chapter. Generally, delusional forms of jealousy are regarded as the most alarming and most dangerous, since there is no way of reasoning the individual out of his mistaken belief.

One thing must be said here. In many cases of delusional jealousy the accusations are totally untrue and the person who is accused is utterly bewildered by what is happening. There are some occasions, however, on which the partner has actually been unfaithful. The morbidly jealous individual may or may not actually know this but the accusations are still made in a totally unreasonable way. One can see what a frightening situation this will be for the accused person and what a delicate problem it may pose for the therapist, trying to estimate at what point the recriminations go beyond the bounds of reason in a context which is already unreasonable, and knowing how best to handle the dilemma.

When is jealousy pathological?

If jealousy is part of the human condition then its expression has to be regarded in general as 'normal', even if sometimes reprehensible. It is part of the burden we carry from our animal past in which exclusion of rivals and protection of one's own clan was vital for survival. In civilised circumstances we can accept the existence of jealousy but generally prefer that its overt manifestations are kept under control. The decision about when jealousy becomes pathological therefore has to be largely a social one: in many societies, for example, there is still a lingering acknowledgement of the *crime passionel*, the crime which is to some extent thought excusable because it is committed out of love – very often jealous love. In most societies the excusability is one way: a jealous man who murders his wife's lover is more likely to be forgiven than a jealous wife who commits a similar offence.

In normal jealousy, no matter how strong or violent it may be, there is usually an explanation and even if there is serious misunderstanding on the part of the jealous individual, his or her reaction can be viewed as a comprehensible response to a provocative situation. In pathological jealousy, whether it be 'neurotic' or 'psychotic' and whether it be expressed openly or not, it has been suggested that the following features are distinctive (Cobb, 1984):

(1) The jealous thinking and its associated behaviour are unreasonable, both in the form which they take and the intensity with which they are demonstrated.
(2) No matter how convinced the jealous individual is of the other person's guilt, the evidence is dubious to other people, although, as has just been noted, the situation is not always a straightforward one to the observer.
(3) A recognisable psychiatric disorder may be present which could initiate or aggravate emotions of jealousy.
(4) The jealous individual often (but not always) has relevant premorbid personality characteristics of jealousy, over-possessiveness and suspiciousness.
(5) The jealousy lasts unduly long: because it is pathological it must always remain uncertain and continue to generate further jealousy. (As LaRochefoucald so succinctly said, 'Jealousy feeds upon suspicion, and it turns into fury or ends as soon as we pass from suspicion to certainty'.)
(6) Pathological jealousy is usually focused with unusual intensity on one specific person and no other.

In addition to these characteristics, the individual's abnormal jealousy is a profound preoccupation which takes up an increasing amount of time. In the 'neurotic' type, which has many features suggestive of obsessive–compulsive mechanisms, there is high awareness of the emotion and sometimes of its irrationality, and irritation at being unable to express it. In the delusional form the person is totally at one with the belief, even when enraged by it, and he or she cannot be convinced by reasoned argument or with contradiction by proof, no matter how overwhelming the latter. Particularly in the jealousy subtype of delusional disorder, the patients' monomaniacal intensity of belief, their ability to produce 'evidence' and their unrelenting pursuit of the victim, are totally abnormal, but because they remain so high-functioning otherwise they may be very persuasive to outsiders that they are in the right. They may sometimes even be able to brainwash their victims into believing that they actually are guilty of infidelity.

The impact of pathological jealousy

Any kind of jealousy, no matter how normal, is a source of anguish to the individual experiencing it, and in the abnormal forms it may well be anguish that goes on night and day: 'And even in our sleep pain that cannot forget falls drop by drop upon the heart . . . ' (Aeschylus). But just as important as its impact on the sufferer is the devastating effect on the sexual partner who is accused of infidelity. Proof of innocence, indignation, righteous anger and protest have no effect and the victim (sometimes also the family) are subjected to escalating emotional assault (Sharma, 1991).

Not uncommonly the person who first presents with serious problems is not the patient, but the partner. He or she is likely to be severely distressed and may become housebound in a vain attempt to avoid accusations of philandering. Sometimes the partner may even attempt suicide in a desperate effort to find relief and this may be when the intolerable domestic situation comes to light. The following case is of just such a presentation.

Case No 7   Delusional disorder, jealousy subtype

A woman of 52 was admitted to hospital after taking an overdose. She had no previous psychiatric history and at first was reluctant to discuss the reason for the suicide attempt. Then she broke down and blurted out a story (later confirmed by her daughter) of constant persecution by her husband for the past two years. Although their relationship had been happy until then, he had developed the unshakable conviction that she was being unfaithful and for these two years he had been incessantly accusing her of infidelity. In recent months his accusations had escalated and he insisted that she was having affairs with many men at work. Even if she got up at night to go to the toilet he would say that she had met a man outside the room, and he had taken to arranging her clothing in certain ways after she went to bed in order to 'prove' that she had slipped out of the house while he was asleep. During the night, when cars passed their home, he was convinced they flashed their headlights in certain ways to make assignations. Although not physically violent to her, his manner had become very threatening and she overdosed because she could no longer tolerate his suspiciousness.

The husband willingly came for interview and he confirmed all his wife had said. He was fully convinced of her guilt although, when pressed, admitted he had no direct proof and agreed that his wife had never been flirtatious. He was distressed by her 'unfaithfulness' but was also distressed at his own behaviour and was very upset by his wife's suicide attempt. He quite readily agreed to accept treatment, although his justification was that he was 'upset' rather than that he had any mental illness.

He was a man of somewhat limited intelligence but a hard worker and good provider. He had been a heavy drinker as a young man, but in his early 40s he had deliberately reduced his alcohol intake and now only drank socially. He had no apparent previous psychiatric history and no significant family history of psychiatric disorder.

On neuroleptic medication, his jealous delusions rapidly settled down and both partners became much happier. He proved to be an extremely compliant patient and over the next six years he took his treatment regularly. On several occasions the dose was tentatively reduced but he himself reported being uneasy because he would begin to be more watchful of his wife, so each time his maintenance dose was increased back to its previous effective level. There was no serious recurrence but the story has an unhappy ending. His wife developed cancer and died: apparently unable to live without her, the patient fatally overdosed on his neuroleptic medication.

In this particular example, physical violence did not occur, but in fact this is an ever-present danger with delusions of jealousy and in a proportion of cases can finally lead to homicide. Some cases of murder, followed by the suicide of the perpetrator, are an outcome of jealous delusions, perhaps especially in women (Fishbain, 1986).

Lay authors are fascinated by morbid jealousy and Othello, of course, is the best-known fictional character with this disorder. Indeed, pathological jealousy is sometimes called the 'Othello syndrome' (Schmeideberg, 1953), but this term is misleading. First, it is used to describe any type of excessive jealousy, especially where there is a tragic outcome, and this lack of precision makes it worthless clinically. Secondly, it certainly should not apply to delusional jealousy since, insofar as we can make a diagnosis in a fictional character, Othello was a man driven to desperation by the evil insinuations of Iago rather than someone who developed spontaneously an erroneous belief about Desdemona.

General aspects of delusional jealousy

We shall shortly discuss the differential diagnosis of pathological jealousy, where it will be emphasized that it can occur in the setting of a number of psychiatric illnesses. Here, we shall look briefly at some of the features which characterize delusional jealousy, whatever the underlying psychiatric disorder.

As has been noted, because the belief is delusional it is accepted by the patient as an absolute and he or she holds to it against all reason or proof. There is usually a good deal of associated irritability, despondency and, at times, aggressiveness which may remain verbal but too often becomes physical. The individual spends an ever-increasing proportion of time searching for 'proof' and the most trivial 'clues' are pounced upon and misinterpreted according to the delusion. The more psychotic the illness, the less rational are the accusations and the victim is put through endless interrogations. However, despite the lack of inherent rationality in the accuser's beliefs, in paranoia/delusional disorder the accusations may sound very convincing and the bewildered victim's protests weak in comparison.

Oddly, when the jealous individual is closely questioned about the extremely pointed charges being made, he or she usually becomes vague on details and falls back on repetitive statements, becoming angry at being quizzed or doubted. It is also strange but true that very often the jealous person avoids actions which might be expected to produce truly unequivocal evidence of the other person's guilt. Whether this is due to fear of failure or to some strange volitional problem related to the illness is not known.

Pathological jealousy is more often described in men but this may be because males have a greater propensity for violence and homicide, which makes their delusion more noticeable. However, pathological jealousy, including delusional jealousy, occurs in both sexes, and the ratio should probably be considered equal until authoritative evidence proves otherwise.

But another possibility why jealousy delusions are more frequently reported in men is because of the long-recognized apparent link with alcohol abuse and, more recently, with abuse of other drugs, especially amphetamines and cocaine (Alarcon, 1980). Michael and colleagues (1995) found that 34 per cent of a group of actively alcoholic male alcoholics showed morbid jealousy: 16 of the 71 (22.5 per cent) appeared to have delusional illnesses and 9 of these had delusions of the jealous type. Soyka (1992) also reports a raised frequency of delusional jealousy in alcoholism and, interestingly, in dementing disorders, including dementia of old age. In clinical practice it is certainly not unusual to find elderly patients with Alzheimer's disease making jealous accusations against partners of many years' standing; one demented patient in the writer's experience began to make unfounded retrospective accusations of infidelity against his wife, who had died several years previously of a long and debilitating illness.

The overall prevalence of morbid jealousy is totally unknown as is the frequency of delusional disorder of the jealous subtype. Crowe and colleagues (1988) remarked that delusional jealousy patients seemed better able than other deluded patients to remain out of hospital and, if so, hospital-based figures must give totally unreliable estimates. Many of the victims live in fear, so it is possible that they will not readily seek help for themselves or the patient who, of course, will absolutely deny being unwell. As domestic violence becomes a less secretive topic in society and as more resources are provided for abused and assaulted spouses and partners, it is probable that more cases of delusional jealousy will be uncovered. And, it should be emphasized, cases of both heterosexual and homosexual delusional jealousy exist and virtually nothing is known of the frequency of the latter.

Family patterns of jealous behaviour have been described and Vauhkonen (1968) suggested the possibility of heritability. A former colleague of the author, Dr. Richard Swinson, has had experience of a patient and her family where morbid jealousy of a nonpsychotic nature has occurred in three successive generations of women with marked features of obsessionality being involved (Swinson, 1981, personal communication). On the whole, if genetic or familial factors are of some importance, it is likely to be in normal jealousy or jealousy of the 'neurotic' type rather than in delusional jealousy. As has been noted elsewhere (see pp.58–59), delusional disorders do not generally seem to run to type in succeeding generations, and Crowe and colleagues (1988) seem to confirm that this is specifically true of those with jealousy delusions.

The jealousy which occurs in delusional disorder may appear gradually or suddenly but, even when the onset is rapid, there is often a considerable prodromal period of increasing uncertainty and rumination which may be analogous to the experience of 'delusional mood' (Wahnstimmung), which is a frequent precursor to actual delusions (see p.30).

The course of normal jealousy depends very much on circumstances, but there will be a tendency towards resolution as the provoking circumstances disappear or the individual realises he/she has lost the struggle to retain the other person. On the other hand, morbid jealousy of neurotic or personality-related type seems in many instances to be very chronic, probably lifelong in some cases. Delusional jealousy is also potentially lifelong but may wax or wane according to the progression of the underlying psychotic illness. The 'purest' form of delusional jealousy, that of paranoia/delusional disorder, used to have the worst prognosis and the most chronic course, but this may have changed as delusional disorder has become more treatable.

The psychopathology of morbid jealousy

This is a contentious and ill-understood area, even though the psychoanalytic literature would lead us to believe that the aetiology of jealousy has been definitively described. Freeman (1990) reviews the writings of Freud, especially his 1922 paper entitled 'some neurotic mechanisms in jealousy, paranoia and homosexuality', in which Freud differentiates between jealousy of the neurotic and of the delusional type. In the former he believed that there was a pre-conscious or unconscious heterosexual wish externalised on to the heterosexual partner, whereas in delusional jealousy he described an unconscious homosexual wish which is externalised on to the heterosexual partner. Although there has been strong theoretical objection to the linking of homosexuality, whether overt or 'latent', to the genesis of paranoia of jealous or any type, this unproven hypothesis continues to masquerade as fact in some writings. An equally unproven theory is that of Melanie Klein (1957) who stated that jealousy derived from early envy, ultimately envy of the mother's breast.

Pao (1969) implicated narcissistic mechanisms in the development of jealousy, and suggested that jealousy was a substitute for, and defence against, full, loving and sexual intimacy with another individual.

All such statements are so general and incapable of experimental proof that they can, at best, be regarded as metaphors in trying to understand the (as yet) ununderstandable and in developing some kind of language with which to communicate with the jealous patient in therapy. It must be stressed that we really know nothing about the psychological origins of jealousy or the nature of its relationship to paranoia/delusional disorder. Coen (1987) shows some welcome frankness when he says that psychoanalytic investigation of delusional jealousy has been hampered because the patient is usually too disturbed: in other words, psychotherapists (including Freud) rarely accept psychotic patients in treatment and therefore have little material on which to hypothesise on delusional features and none to theorise on aetiology.

The differential diagnosis of delusional jealousy

If we are considering a diagnosis of delusional disorder, jealousy subtype, what other conditions must we consider before discarding them in favour of this one? The following list of possibilities should be borne in mind:

(1) Actual marital or sexual problems: as noted, there is always the possibility that the individual's sexual partner has indeed been unfaithful and that the accusations are true. This is only likely to come to the attention of the treating psychiatrist if the jealous patient is receiving attention for a psychiatric illness and his or her accusations emerge: then one has to decide whether the jealousy is 'normal' or is an integral part of that other illness.

(2) Mental handicap: this is sometimes a background factor in jealousy. A simple-minded person may develop a severe 'crush' on someone, perhaps a caregiver, and will have difficulty understanding that the other person's romantic affections lie elsewhere. Or, where a mentally retarded person has entered into a sexual relationship, he or she may become jealous because of inability to understand the partner's motives or behaviour.

(3) Schizophrenia: especially in paranoid schizophrenia the individual may develop severe delusions of all kinds, including jealousy, not uncommonly mixed with some degree of persecutory belief and/or grandiosity.

(4) Major mood disorder: in some depressive episodes of psychotic intensity the delusions may have a content of jealousy, not uncommonly linked to feelings of severe self-worthlessness. Less often, the manic patient may be jealous and irritable and may act out these feelings in a blatant way.

(5) Personality disorders: a wide variety of personality disorders may present with marked jealousy features, most notably paranoid, schizoid, antisocial, borderline, histrionic and narcissistic types.

(6) Obsessive–compulsive disorder: the typical obsessive–compulsive does not display jealousy as a feature of the illness but, on the other hand, so-called 'neurotic' morbid jealousy often appears to have a very marked quality of obsessionality, with the individual being aware of the emotion but unable to suppress it.

(7) Substance abuse: as already mentioned, there appears to be a connection between abuse of alcohol, amphetamines or cocaine and the development of pathological jealousy. The abuse need not be current and indeed in some individuals it may have ceased a considerable time before the symptoms of jealousy appear.

(8) Organic brain disorders: Mooney (1965) pointed out that many types of brain dysfunction may result in pathological jealousy. Other workers, including Flor-Henry (1969) and Cummings (1985), have suggested that left temporal lesions are especially likely to be associated with delusional illness. It is known that some cases of epileptic psychosis are accompanied by delusions of jealousy.

(9) Sexual dysfunction: if there are persistent sexual difficulties and one partner becomes concerned that the other may seek satisfaction elsewhere, then jealousy may arise. Sometimes the dysfunction is physical (for example, as a long-term complication of alcohol abuse – a doubly loaded situation for jealousy to appear), or it may be related to persistent psychosexual difficulties between partners.

(10) Delusional disorder, jealousy subtype: if the disorder we are faced with consists of a monodelusional presentation in which there is an encapsulated delusional system whose predominant theme is jealousy, with relative sparing of the rest of the personality, and if we have carefully excluded the other possibilities mentioned above, it is likely that we are dealing with paranoia/delusional disorder.

In any diagnostic process in psychiatry we have to carry out careful history-taking and this may not be easy in a high-functioning delusional person who does not accept that he has a mental illness and who resents having to talk to a psychiatrist. The situation is made doubly difficult because it may be impossible to obtain an adequate collateral history when the partner is terrorised by the patient's threats. In a situation like this it would be ideal to admit the patient to hospital and observe his/her mental state and behaviour there, but often that is only possible when an offence – an assault on the partner, for example – has occurred and the patient is committed, involuntarily.

Forensic complications

As discussed, the frequency of pathological jealousy of any type is unknown, so the frequency of assault on the jealousy victim is equally unknown, but the numbers must be considerable. Often, if physical abuse in a relationship comes to light it takes some time to appreciate that in a proportion of cases it is due to delusional jealousy. It is important to bear this possibility in mind at all times because of the chance of escalation to severe violence and murder. In two series of cases of delusional jealousy, the frequency of murder by deluded individuals was 4 per cent (Shepherd, 1961) and 2 per cent (Retterstøl, 1967), respectively. In a series of criminally insane murderers, Mowat (1966) found that 12 per cent of the males and 15 per cent of the females had killed because of jealousy.

As was noted earlier, attempted suicide and even suicide by a desperate victim have been recorded. In other cases, the deluded person has committed homicide and then committed suicide (Fishbain, 1986).

In a situation where a physician has recognized the presence of pathological jealousy and believes there is imminent danger to the partner, he or she has a duty to warn and protect the latter. This may involve divulging confidential information to the victim and/or to the authorities, and in some cases may require involuntary committal of the delusional person to an institution. This latter can be very difficult to achieve legally or to maintain, in a person who retains a degree of social functioning and who has sufficient insight to conceal the abnormality temporarily when faced with law enforcement measures. Not only that, being 'paranoid' he may also be potentially litigious and it may take some degree of moral courage to deal with such a situation. However, there is nothing worse than to have failed to act on one's reasonable suspicions and to discover that murder, perhaps preventable, has taken place.

In Chapter 5, in which we deal with Erotomania, the phenomenon of stalking, usually of females by predatory males, is discussed. This kind of behaviour can be related to a variety of possible psychopathologies in the stalker, only one of which is erotomania. It seems likely that a proportion of cases may also be due to delusions of jealousy but, whereas in erotomania the victim has no idea who the man is, in jealous stalking it is usually the sexual partner who is the victim and that person is acutely aware who the perpetrator is.

Treatment and prognosis of delusional disorder, jealousy subtype

Each of the jealousy-associated disorders we have mentioned has its own treatment. For example, cases in which marital problems are predominant and conditions related to personality disorders and to sexual dysfunctions may be best approached with counselling, psychotherapy and cognitive behavioural modification (Bishay, Petersen and Tarrier, 1989; Tarrier and colleagues, 1990), in addition to any physical treatments which may be required for the sexual disorder. In the so-called 'neurotic' type of morbid jealousy there has been a decided improvement in outlook in recent years, especially if the disorder has obsessional features. In these cases, there have been a number of reports of successful treatment with specific serotonin reuptake inhibitor (SSRI) antidepressants (Lane, 1990; Gross, 1991; Stein, Hollander and Josephson, 1994).

Schizophrenia and major mood disorders should respond to neuroleptics and antidepressants. Persistent substance abuse requires detoxification followed by prolonged counselling and involvement in self-help programmes. If delusional jealousy still persists after the substance abuse has ceased, neuroleptic treatment should be initiated.

If the established diagnosis is that of delusional disorder, jealousy subtype, treatment with a neuroleptic is also indicated but is sometimes very difficult with an insightless, resistant patient. One must spend considerable time trying to obtain the individual's trust and persuading him or her that treatment is required; after a time it will be, not too uncommonly, reluctantly accepted in these circumstances and if one can persist with an adequate dosage of the appropriate neuroleptic, tension will defuse after a week or two and then the delusion will diminish, and may even disappear.

At the risk of appearing repetitive, one needs to reiterate that many psychiatrists still hold to the outdated idea that delusional disorder, because it was formerly paranoia which was regarded as untreatable, is inaccessible to neuroleptic treatment. This is quite false, and although there are, as yet, no scientific drug trials reported in relation to delusional jealousy, there are a number of anecdotal accounts suggesting that good to excellent results may be obtained with the use of low dose pimozide, as in other forms of delusional disorder (Dorian, 1979; Pollock, 1982; Munro, 1984; Byrne and Yatham, 1989; Iruela and colleagues, 1989; Cooper, 1991). For further details of treatment of delusional disorder, see Chapter 13.

Conclusion

Psychiatry is frequently criticised for its excessive use of jargon and certainly, when esoteric terms are used mainly for effect, they may serve to confuse issues rather than to clarify them. However, we also suffer from the frequent use of lay terms which have been given some kind of technical nuance, though not necessarily with any clear definition of the new meaning. The word 'jealousy' is too often taken for granted even in technical writings and the reader has to surmise whether the author means the normal human emotion or some exaggeration of that, or whether pathological jealousy is implied and, if so, which subtype of that. Such lack of definitions makes any description inscrutable and renders research impossible.

Having recognized jealousy as a central feature of a patient's psychopathology we have to resist the temptation to see that as the illness. It is the content of a belief within a disorder whose form is what matters. So, jealousy can be a content of delusional disorder, major mood disorder, obsessive–compulsive disorder or narcissistic personality disorder, as well as others and, for all we know, may arise for entirely different reasons in each of these illnesses. Specific description of the phenomenon and equally specific attribution to an illness (if present) are therefore both necessary.

During the time that paranoia/delusional disorder was in abeyance as a widely used diagnosis, many cases of its jealousy subtype were regarded as schizophrenic. There are therefore very few recent references in the literature specifically relating to delusional disorder with jealousy symptoms. No doubt this will change as knowledge about delusional disorder in general becomes more widely disseminated. In the meantime, the reader is advised to cast a highly critical eye on any publication concerning 'pathological jealousy', before accepting its assertions.

References

Alarcon, R. (1980). El sindrome de Otelo. *Acta Psiquiat. Psicol. Am. Lat.* **26**: 318–326.
Bishay, N.R., Petersen, N. and Tarrier, N. (1989). An uncontrolled study of cognitive therapy for morbid jealousy. *Br. J. Psychiat* **154**: 386–389.
Byrne, A. and Yatham, L. (1989). Pimozide in pathological jealousy. *Br. J. Psychiat.* **155**: 249–251.
Cobb, J. (1984). Morbid jealousy. In *Contemporary Psychiatry*, ed. S. Crown, pp. 68–79. London: Butterworths.
Coen, S.J. (1987). Pathological jealousy. *Int. J. Psycho-Anal.* **68**: 99–108.
Cooper, S.A. (1991). Long-term prognosis of pathological jealousy in an elderly man treated with pimozide. *Psychiat. Pract.*, Winter: 9–10.
Crowe, R.R., Clarkson, C., Tsai, M. and Wilson, R. (1988). Delusional disorder: jealous and nonjealous types. *Eur. Arch. Psychiatr. Neurol. Sci.* **237**: 179–183.

Cummings, J.L. (1985). Organic delusions: phenomenology, anatomical correlations, and review. *Br. J. Psychiat.* **146**: 184–197.

Dorian, B.J. (1979). Monosymptomatic hypochondriacal psychosis. *Can. J. Psychiat.* **24**: 377 (letter).

Fishbain, D.B. (1986). Suicide pacts and homicide. *Am. J. Psychiat.* **143**: 1319–1320 (letter).

Flor-Henry, P. (1969). Schizophrenic-like reactions and affective psychosis associated with temporal lobe epilepsy: etiological factors. *Am. J. Psychiat.* **126**: 400–404.

Freeman, T. (1990). Psychoanalytical aspects of morbid jealousy in women. *Br. J. Psychiat.* **156**: 68–72.

Gross, M.D. (1991). Treatment of pathological jealousy by fluoxetine. *Am. J. Psychiat.* **148**: 683–684 (letter).

Iruela, L.M., Gilaberte, I., Caballero, L. and Oliveros, S.C. (1989). Pathological jealousy and pimozide. *Br. J. Psychiat.* **155**: 749 (letter).

Klein, M. (1957). Envy and gratitude In *The Writings of Melanie Klein*, Vol. 3, pp. 176–235. London: Hogarth Press.

Lane, R.D. (1990). Successful fluoxetine treatment of pathologic jealousy. *J. Clin. Psychiat.* **51**: 345–346.

Mathes, E.W., Adams, H.E. and Davies, R.M. (1985). Jealousy: loss of relationship rewards, loss of self-esteem, depression, anxiety, and anger. *J. Personal. Social Psychol.* **48**:1552–1561.

Michael, A., Mirza, S., Mirza, K.A.H., Babu, V.S. and Vithayathil, E. (1995). Morbid jealousy in alcoholism. *Br. J. Psychiat.* **167**: 668–672.

Mooney, H.B. (1965). Pathological jealousy and psychochemotherapy. *Br. J. Psychiat.* **111**: 1023–1042.

Mowat, R.R. (1966). *Morbid Jealousy and Murder.* London: Tavistock Publications.

Mullen, P.E. and Martin, J. (1994). Jealousy: a community study. *Br. J. Psychiat.* **164**: 35–43.

Munro, A. (1989). When does jealousy become a psychiatric problem? *Can. J. Diag.* **6**: 123–129.

Munro, A. (1984). Excellent response of pathologic jealousy to pimozide. *Can. Med. Ass. J.* **131**: 852–853 (letter).

Pao, P.N. (1969). Pathological jealousy. *Psychoanal. Quart.* **38**: 616–638.

Pollock, B.G. (1982). Successful treatment of pathological jealousy with pimozide. *Can. J. Psychiat.* **27**: 86–87 (letter).

Retterstøl, N. (1967). Jealousy–paranoiac psychoses. *Acta Psychiat. Scand.* **43**: 75–107.

Schmeideberg, M. (1953). Some aspects of jealousy and of feeling hurt. *Psychoanal. Rev.* **40**: 1–16.

Seeman, M. (1979). Pathological jealousy. *Psychiatry* **42**: 351–361.

Sahrma, V.P. (1991). *Insane Jealousy*, pp. 29–72. Cleveland, Tennessee: Mind Publications.

Shepherd, M. (1961). Morbid jealousy: some clinical and social aspects of a psychiatric syndrome. *J. Ment. Sci.* **107**: 687–753.

Soyka, M. (1992). Delusional jealousy in psychiatric disorders of later life. *Int. J. Geriat. Psychiat.* **7**: 539–542.

Soyka, M., Naber, G. and Völcker, A. (1991). Prevalence of delusional jealousy in different psychiatric disorders: an analysis of 93 cases. *Br. J. Psychiat.* **158**: 549–553.

Stein, D.J., Hollander, E. and Josephson, S.C. (1994). Serotonin reuptake
    blockers for the treatment of obsessional jealousy. *J. Clin. Psychiat.* **55**:
    30–33.
Tarrier, N., Beckett, R., Harwood, S. and Bishay, N. (1990). Morbid jealousy: a
    review and cognitive–behavioural formulation. *Br. J. Psychiat.* **157**:
    319–326.
Vauhkonen, K. (1968). On the pathogenesis of morbid jealousy. *Acta Psychiat.
    Scand.* Suppl. 202.

5

Delusional disorder, erotomanic subtype

In erotomania, an individual has the fixed, unfounded belief that another person is deeply in love with him or her. The condition is usually regarded as delusional although a small number of cases may be non-delusional (Meloy, 1990). In some instances the imagined lover does not exist and is a 'phantom' (Seeman, 1978) but more generally is a real person who is unaware of the situation. He or she is often socially unattainable to the erotomanic sufferer and rarely has had close personal contact with the latter; and, in fact, frequently does not know he or she exists.

During the seventeenth century this 'amor insanus' was differentiated from nymphomania, which is the insatiable lust in a female for sexual intercourse, so its existence has been known for a very long time. As will be mentioned, until relatively recently erotomania was thought of as occurring almost exclusively in females, but is now known also to affect males.

Erotomania is frequently associated with the name of de Clérambault, a French psychiatrist who described the condition in some detail (de Clérambault, 1942). But in fact, as Segal (1989) has pointed out, Emil Kraepelin (1921) had already written about an erotomanic variety of paranoia much earlier and in this chapter it is his description of monodelusional erotomania which is emphasized.

de Clérambault, to his credit, distinguished a 'pure' or 'primary' erotomania (more or less approximating to Kraepelin's paranoia) from symptomatic erotomanias which could occur as part of other psychiatric disorders. Because of paranoia's virtual demise as a recognized diagnostic entity in the middle of the twentieth century and because, until recently, very few cases of erotomania were described in the literature, a great deal of confusion arose about the nature of the disorder, with some authorities insisting that it was always symptomatic of other conditions and denying that erotomania could exist as a primary illness (Ellis and Mellsop, 1985;

Signer, 1991). In recent years, more cases have been published showing that both primary and secondary forms exist, implying that it can be a syndrome as well as an illness in its own right. In 1987, DSMIIIR included primary erotomania as a subtype of delusional disorder and this author can certainly attest to having seen a number of patients in which this diagnosis was the most appropriate. This form of erotomania comes nearest to being a specific illness in its own right, although one should hasten to add that it is identical to other subtypes of delusional disorder, except in the specific nature of its delusional content.

When erotomania is recognized, careful history-taking and differential diagnosis are essential to ensure appropriate treatment. Nowadays, cases of erotomania are being described with increasing frequency, and some of them have legal significance as well as clinical interest. As the number of case descriptions grows, the proportion of men with the diagnosis becomes more significant. Most cases are heterosexual in nature, but several descriptions of homosexual erotomania have appeared, affecting both males and females (Lovett Doust and Christie, 1978; Peterson and Davis, 1985; Dunlop, 1988).

The following are the characteristics generally demonstrated by patients with erotomania (Taylor, Mahendra and Gunn, 1983; Ellis and Mellsop, 1985):

(1) The patient has the unshakeable conviction that he/she is loved by a specific individual who is often of higher social standing and sometimes is a prominent figure or even a celebrity.
(2) Although the other person has had little (or absolutely no) previous contact with the patient, the latter usually believes that the other initiated the relationship.
(3) The patient usually has strongly erotic feelings towards the other person, although sometimes the 'relationship' is regarded as platonic.
(4) The other person is usually unattainable in some way, for example because of marital status or high social visibility. In many cases the patient never makes any attempt to contact the love-object, often writing letters but not mailing them, or buying presents but never sending them. Even when given a chance to make real contact, the patient will frequently avoid doing so and will devise spurious explanations to account for this.
(5) In those individuals who do make contact with the other person, reasons are found to explain the 'paradoxical' (i.e. rejecting) behaviour which is naturally shown by the latter. In some instances, there may be

anger about this perceived rejection associated with acting out behaviour (see below).

(6) Sometimes the other person is believed to protect, watch over or follow the patient and all kinds of behaviours are misinterpreted as evidence of passionate interest.

(7) The onset of erotomania may be sudden or gradual.

(8) Hallucinations may be present and some individuals with tactile hallucinations may believe that they have been visited by a lover during the night, a phenomenon sometimes known as the 'incubus syndrome' (Raschka, 1979).

(9) When the case is one of 'pure' or 'primary' erotomania, the accompanying features are those of delusional disorder as described in Chapter 2. That is, it is a monodelusional disorder with relative preservation of normal personality features and often some capacity to remain functional in society. In these cases the patient not infrequently is able to conceal the abnormal belief from other people (Munro, 1989). Thought disorder is virtually absent outside the delusional system.

The differential diagnosis of erotomania

When an individual is recognized as having erotomanic delusions, the following disorders must be considered:

(1) Delusional disorder, erotomanic subtype.

(2) Schizophrenia, especially of the paranoid type. Here, there will usually be other delusions with a variety of themes, hallucinations and relatively widespread thought disorder. The personality is less well preserved and obvious abnormalities of behaviour may occur (Hayes and O'Shea, 1985; El-Assra, 1989; Gillett, Eminson and Hassanyeh, 1990).

(3) Major mood disorders. Erotomania has been noted in association with unipolar and bipolar affective disorders (Remington and Book, 1984; Rudden, Sweeney and Frances, 1990; Wood and Poe, 1990), and there is a description based on one case which suggests that it can appear as a variant of pathological mourning (Evans, Jeckel and Slott, 1982).

(4) Various organic brain disorders. There have been descriptions of erotomania occurring in epilepsy, as part of the after-effects of head injury and among the late effects of substance abuse (Lovett Doust and Christie, 1978; El-Gaddal, 1989). It has also been observed in senile dementia (Drevets and Rubin, 1987; Carrier, 1990), and apparently as a side effect of certain therapeutic drugs including oral contraceptives

and steroids (Lovett Doust and Christie, 1978). Signer and Cummings (1987) have suggested that abnormalities of the left temporal lobe may be particularly likely to cause symptoms of erotomania.

(5) Mental handicap. Collacott (1987) and Ghaziuddin and Tsai (1991) have reported erotomanic delusions in mentally retarded individuals. There is no reason why such persons cannot have delusions associated with a superimposed psychiatric illness, but it is possible that part of their erotomania may be due to a simple person's misunderstanding of another individual's intentions. However, in this context, one must be aware that mentally handicapped patients can sometimes be taken advantage of sexually by helpers or relatives, and that sexually-laden remarks made by the patient about others may have had a basis in fact.

(6) Delusional misidentification syndrome (DMS). Erotomania has been described in association with DMS in a small number of cases (Signer and Isbister, 1987; Wright, Young and Hellawell, 1993). This is interesting in view of the thesis to be put forward later in this book (see Chapter 9), that DMS should be included in the official description of delusional disorders.

(7) Shared psychotic disorder (*folie à deux*). A sharing of the erotomanic beliefs with another individual (not the victim), and acceptance of these as truth by that individual, has been described (Pearce, 1972). This is hardly surprising since *folie à deux* has been shown to be relatively common in delusional disorder (Munro, 1982).

(8) Non-delusional erotomanic beliefs. These have already been touched upon, and it does appear that certain people may have very powerful erotomanic emotions which are in the nature of over-valued ideas rather than delusions (Seeman, 1978; Evans, Jeckel and Slott, 1982). It is important to make this distinction because, in such cases, psychotherapy rather than medication may be indicated.

Sex distribution of erotomania

In the earlier part of the twentieth century, Kretschmer (1927) introduced the concept of 'the erotic self-reference psychosis of old maids', but with a strong emphasis on certain conflicting premorbid personality traits such as over-sensitivity and vulnerability on the one hand and 'priggishness' and prudery on the other. Other workers have not found convincing evidence of such a constellation of symptoms (for example Retterstøl, 1967), but the influence of Kretschmer and other authorities, especially perhaps Hart (1921) promoted the stereotype of erotomania as a disorder occurring mainly in middle-aged or elderly spinsters, living lonely and embittered lives and obtaining their only sexual satisfaction through vicarious erotic delusional feelings towards an imaginary lover.

In fact, erotomania occurs in both sexes, as de Clérambault himself (1942) had certainly realised, and Goldstein (1986) has written extensively about this. The relative frequency of erotomania in the two sexes is unknown, either in the delusional disorder subtype or as a symptom of other psychiatric illnesses, but the phenomenon is certainly not uncommon in males. What has come to be realised is that erotomanic males are much more likely to act out their delusional fantasies, sometimes dangerously.

Case No. 8   Delusional disorder, erotomanic subtype

A 42-year-old unmarried bank teller had lived with his widowed mother all his life. He was regarded as a hard worker, but he mixed very little with fellow workers and appeared to have virtually no social life. He did not drink or smoke. His father had died young and he did not remember him. At the age of 40 he lost his mother who had a stroke and died after a short illness. He appeared very dejected and took several weeks off work, then returned as quiet and uncommunicative as ever.

On most days of the week, a young woman who worked in a nearby business came into the bank to deposit money. The patient had often served her at the counter but showed no especial interest in her. Then, one day about four months after his mother's death, he was taking money from her and he suddenly became aware that she was looking at him in a very intense way. He became distressed but managed to finish the transaction and then rushed to the staff room, where it took him several minutes to calm down. He was upset by his reaction and could not explain it. That night in bed he had an erection and a nocturnal emission and he suddenly 'realised' that this young woman was intensely in love with him. He felt both panicky and exultant at this thought.

He was apprehensive about going to work the next day, but once there he began to look forward to seeing the woman again and thereafter always tried to make sure that he served her. With each visit he became increasingly convinced that she was transmitting cryptic messages to him by tone of voice, movements, attitudes, etc. She did not make any open declaration of her feelings but he 'knew' this was because she did not want the other tellers to realise the intensity of her passion. He felt it was his duty to respect her silence but tried to indicate wordlessly to her that he understood. One day she accidentally left behind a scrap of paper on which she had written some words – presumably related to her work. He surreptitiously took it home, 'decoded' its message, and thereafter used it as a sexual fetish, masturbating while reading the writing on it.

He took to writing letters to her but never sent them. Then, after work he began to hang around her place of work, following her home, but always taking care she never saw him. Nevertheless, he would be convinced that when she came in next day she was communicating her approval of his interest in her. After a time, virtually all his spare moments were taken up with fantasising about her or following her. One weekend, a male cousin from another city visited the woman's family home and took her out for dinner. The patient shadowed the couple and as they emerged from the restaurant he suddenly went berserk, flailing at the man (who was much bigger than he) and screaming at the woman that she was unfaithful and a slut, and that he would kill her.

He was soon overpowered and arrested. His conversation was so bizarre that he was remanded for a psychiatric opinion. Under observation conditions he settled down over a period of several days, becoming polite, quiet and apparently rational, except that he insisted that he had been motivated by the young woman's provocative behaviour. She was able to convince the authorities that she was completely bewildered by his accusations. A diagnosis of delusional disorder, erotomanic type, was eventually made, as the patient's abnormal belief system remained fixed. No features of mood disorder or schizophrenia were noted. He was offered neuroleptic treatment and, rather surprisingly, accepted it. Over the next four weeks he appeared to lose interest in the young woman but, when questioned, would still say that she had provoked him. After three months of treatment he returned to work, but to a different branch of the bank. His behaviour is quiet and inoffensive. One year later he continues to take a maintenance dose of neuroleptic and attends his psychiatrist for review: he has proved inaccessible to psychotherapy. He does not ever mention the woman.

Forensic aspects

In general, women do not flamboyantly act out their erotomanic delusions, although a well-known American film of the 1970s, *Play Misty for Me*, describes in fictional terms the dangerous outcome of erotomania occurring in a female. Less dramatic but nonetheless disturbing instances do sometimes occur in real life, to the annoyance, alarm and distress of the object of the deluded individual's attention; nowadays, when male professionals are under so much moral pressure to guard against inappropriate sexual behaviour towards clients, it can be devastating if a deluded woman publicly declares that a doctor, a counsellor, a university teacher or someone else has been demonstrating strong erotic feelings towards her. If the deluded individual has a nondeteriorated personality, totally believes her own story, and presents her claims as vehemently and persistently as such people do, it may be almost impossible to get the public to believe that what she is saying is untrue. Real unrequited love is bad enough: delusional unrequited love can be impossible.

Taylor, Mahendra and Gunn (1983) studied a group of males charged with antisocial behaviour, including persistent unwelcomed importuning of women, and were able to identify cases of erotomania amongst these. Often they were initially diagnosed as schizophrenic but closer examination sometimes suggested the presence of paranoia/delusional disorder. The same researchers noted that several patients exhibited quite grandiose behaviours, a common feature of delusional disorder which makes it especially difficult to engage in logical discussion with the person about his false belief or to persuade him to change his behaviour. None of these particular cases had behaved violently towards their victims but their unremitting harassment often caused the women involved to feel threatened.

Goldstein (1987) has described cases of severely aggressive, erotomanic behaviour in males, some of whom gained widespread public notoriety. One of these was the young man who attempted to assassinate Ronald Reagan when the latter was President of the United States, apparently believing that this would gain the attention of a well known female film star, towards whom he entertained erotic delusional feelings. Amongst the other cases Goldstein describes, murder, serious assault, kidnapping, and severe harassment occurred. In these individuals the underlying diagnoses were varied but mostly fell within the categories of delusional disorder or paranoid schizophrenia. Goldstein proposes that the changing role of women in society and their higher public profile may act as a stimulus to male erotomania, possibly making the phenomenon more common, but that is hypothetical.

We have no idea of the true frequency of erotomania in all its forms and at present we can only speculate whether it is actually occurring more often or whether it is being recognized more accurately. However, what certainly seems to be becoming alarmingly more frequent is the phenomenon of 'stalking', usually of women by men, and some of these instances are undoubtedly the result of erotomanic delusions (Zona, Sharma and Lane, 1993). The severe impact of stalking on the victims is well described by Pathé and Mullen (1997).

Course and prognosis

The 'pure' or monosymptomatic form of erotomania is the one which usually corresponds with the diagnosis of paranoia/delusional disorder. In the past this has been regarded as unremitting and associated with a poor prognosis but there is now early evidence that, analogous to other subtypes of delusional disorder, the condition may respond well to neuroleptic treatment. As noted in Chapter 13, there is some evidence that pimozide may be especially effective (Munro, O'Brien and Ross, 1985), usually in a daily dose not exceeding 4–6 mg. in most cases.

When erotomania is a symptom of another psychiatric illness such as major mood disorder, schizophrenia or some form of dementia, the course of the phenomenon is that of the parent illness and the prognosis depends on the natural history and adequate treatment of that illness. As has already been noted, it is also important to take into account the possible presence of mental handicap and to consider that, at least in some cases, erotomania may be nondelusional in nature. All of this emphasizes, as always, the need for complete and detailed history-taking and mental status examination as well as careful physical examination. Unfortunately, as we already know, patients with delusional disorder are not always prepared to be co-operative in such investigations.

In special circumstances, as for example in the forensic psychiatric field, where repeated harassment of one person by another, assault of a female by a male, or statements about alleged sexual feelings or behaviours have occurred, great care must be taken with assessment. If the perpetrator has a subtle delusional illness, the facts may be very difficult to tease out and his certainty may, as has been noted, in some ways seem more convincing than the victim's bewilderment and denial. Good collateral information is of the essence here and the person doing the assessment should be aware that professionals in the past have themselves been drawn into a kind of *folie à deux* situation when they have come to believe uncritically in the statements of a highly persuasive paranoiac, as well as being influenced by implied or overt threats of litigation. Accept this author's word that this can sometimes be a very difficult and delicate area through which to pick one's way.

Conclusion

Erotomania may seem an esoteric topic: traditionally an illness occurring mainly in a small number of elderly, love-sick maiden ladies who rarely bother anyone with their delusions. If this were true, it would nevertheless still be worth trying to identify and help such unfortunate people, since any kind of delusional disorder is a wretched affliction. But evidence is accumulating that the disorder in its various forms occurs much more frequently than was realised and that it may be a not inconsiderable cause of harassing, potentially dangerous, or even murderous behaviour in our current social environment.

Identification of cases may be difficult and the secret sufferers who never declare themselves may not be identified. However, we are beginning to be aware of certain high risk groups of individuals which may contain significant numbers of erotomanics, namely 'stalkers', men who persistently harass or assault women with whom they have no obvious connection, and 'unrequited lovers' who are excessively strident and persistent in the accusations they publicly make against the other person. Therefore, be particularly aware of delusional disorder, in this context particularly the erotomanic subtype, and know something of its psychopathology and appropriate treatment.

References

Carrier, L. (1990). Erotomania and senile dementia. *Am. J. Psychiat.* **147**: 1982 (letter).

De Clérambault, C.G. (1942). *Les Psychoses Passionnelles, Oeuvre Psychiatrique.* Paris: Presses Universitaires.

Collacott, R.A. (1987). Erotomanic delusions in mentally handicapped patients: two case reports. *J. Ment. Defic. Res.* **31**: 87–92.

Diagnostic and Statistical Manual of Mental Disorders, 3rd edn revised (DSMIIIR). Washington, DC: American Psychiatric Association.

Drevets, W.C. and Rubin, E.H. (1987). Erotomania and senile dementia of Alzheimer type. *Br. J. Psychiat.* **151**: 400–402.

Dunlop, J.L. (1988). Does erotomania exist between women? *Br. J. Psychiat.* **153**: 830–833.

El-Assra, A. (1989). Erotomania in a Saudi woman. *Br. J. Psychiat.* **155**: 553–555.
El-Gaddal, Y.Y. (1989). De Clérambault's syndrome (erotomania) in organic delusional syndrome. *Br. J. Psychiat.* **154**: 714–716.
Ellis, P. and Mellsop, G. (1985). De Clérambault's syndrome –a nosological entity? *Br. J. Psychiat.* **146**: 90–95.
Evans, D.L., Jeckel, L.L. and Slott, N.E. (1982). Erotomania: a variant of pathological mourning. *Bull. Menninger Clin.* **46**: 507–520.
Ghaziuddin, M. and Tsai, L. (1991). Depression-dependent erotomanic delusions in a mentally handicapped woman. *Br. J. Psychiat.* **158**: 127–129.
Gillett, T., Eminson, S.R. and Hassanyeh, F. (1990). Primary and secondary erotomania: clinical characteristics and follow-up. *Acta Psychiat. Scand.* **82**: 65–69.
Goldstein, R.L. (1986). Erotomania in men. *Am. J. Psychiat.* **143**: 802 (letter).
Goldstein, R.L. (1987). More forensic romances: de Clérambault's syndrome in men. *Bull. Am. Acad. Psychiat. Law* **15**: 267–274.
Hart, B. (1921). *The Psychology of Insanity*. Cambridge: Cambridge University Press.
Hayes, M. and O'Shea, B. (1985). Erotomania in Schneider-positive schizophrenia: a case report. *Br. J. Psychiat.* **146**: 661–663.
Kraepelin, E. (1921). *Manic-Depressive Insanity and Paranoia*. Transl. R.M. Barclay, (1976). New York: Arno Press.
Kretschmer, E. (1927). *Der sensitive Beziehungswahn*, 2nd edn. Berlin: Springer.
Lovett Doust, J.W. and Christie, H. (1978). The pathology of love: some clinical variants of de Clérambault's syndrome. *Soc. Sci. Med.* **12**: 99–106.
Meloy, J.R. (1990). Nondelusional or borderline erotomania. *Am. J. Psychiat.* **147**: 820 (letter).
Munro, A. (1982). *Delusional Hypochondriasis*. Clarke Institute of Psychiatry Monograph No. 5. Toronto: Clarke Institute of Psychiatry.
Munro, A. (1989). Defining the diagnosis of erotomania. *Can. J. Diagn.* **6**: 115–123.
Munro, A., O'Brien, J.V. and Ross, D. (1985). Two cases of 'pure' or 'primary' erotomania successfully treated with pimozide. *Can. J. Psychiat.* **30**: 619–622.
Pathé, M. and Mullen, P.E. (1997). The impact of stalkers on their victims. *Br. J. Psychiat.* **170**: 12–17.
Pearce, A. (1972). De Clérambault's syndrome associated with folie à deux. *Br. J. Psychiat.* **121**: 116–117 (letter).
Peterson, G.A. and Davis, G.L. (1985). A case of homosexual erotomania. *J. Clin. Psychiat.* **46**: 448–449.
Raschka, L.B. (1979). The incubus syndrome, a variant of erotomania. *Can. J. Psychiat.* **24**: 549–553.
Remington, G. and Book, H. (1984). Case report of de Clérambault's syndrome, bipolar affective disorder and response to lithium. *Am. J. Psychiat.* **141**: 1285–1287.
Retterstøl, N. (1967). Erotic self-reference psychosis in old maids. *Acta Psychiat. Scand.* **43**: 347–359.
Rudden, M., Sweeney, J. and Frances, A. (1990). Diagnosis and clinical course of erotomanic and other delusional patients. *Am. J. Psychiat.* **147**: 625–628.
Seeman, M.V. (1978). Delusional loving. *Arch. Gen. Psychiat.* **35**: 1265–1267.
Segal, J.H. (1989). Erotomania revisited: from Kraepelin to DSMIIIR. *Am. J. Psychiat.* **146**: 1261–1266.

Signer, S.F. (1991). Erotomania. *Am. J. Psychiat.* **148**: 1276 (letter).

Signer, S.F. and Cummings, J.L. (1987). De Clérambault's syndrome in organic affective disorder: two cases. *Br. J. Psychiat.* **151**: 404–407.

Signer, S.F. and Isbister, S.R. (1987). Capgras syndrome, de Clérambault's syndrome, and folie à deux. *Br. J. Psychiat.* **151**: 402–404.

Taylor, P., Mahendra, B. and Gunn, J. (1983). Erotomania in males. *Psychol. Med.* **13**: 645–650.

Wood, B.E. and Poe, R.O. (1990). Diagnosis and classification of erotomania. *Am. J. Psychiat.* **147**: 1388–1389 (letter).

Wright, S., Young, A.W. and Hellawell, D.J. (1993). Fregoli delusion and erotomania. *J. Neurol. Neurosurg. Psychiat.* **56**: 322–323 (letter).

Zona, M.A., Sharma, K.K. and Lane, J. (1993). A comparative study of erotomanic and obsessional subjects in a forensic sample. *J. Forens. Sci. JFSCA* **38**: 894–903.

6
Delusional disorder, persecutory/litigious and grandiose subtypes

Persecutory and litigious presentations

Since the archetype of paranoia/delusional disorder is the individual who is convinced that he or she is being persecuted or harmed, and since many people believe that this is the most common form of delusional disorder, one might expect an extensive literature on the phenomenology of persecutory delusions. Certainly, that forms the basis of psychoanalytic theorising on the origin of paranoia (see Chapter 1) but, strangely, despite many references to the subject, there has been remarkably little development of these theories and virtually no systematic study on the topic. Attributions are usually to unsubstantiated hypotheses and eventually refer to anecdotal case analyses.

Nowadays, the neo-Kraepelinian descriptions of delusional disorder in DSMIV (1994) and ICD10 (1992–93) apply equally to each of the subtypes, so a patient with a persecutory subtype would, by definition, have a relatively encapsulated delusional system and a well-preserved personality, the illness being chronic and relatively unremitting. The persecutory beliefs are often associated with querulousness, irritability and anger, and the individual who acts out his anger may be assaultive at times and even homicidal. In expressing his feelings thus, the motivation for violence may be predominantly either a belief that he is defending himself or may be a desire for revenge. As will be mentioned (see pp.138–139), this behaviour may have some important legal repercussions.

Until recently, the definition of delusional disorder emphasized a single, almost exclusive theme (e.g. persecutory, erotomanic, etc.) in every case, although experience indicated that there were often overtones of suspiciousness, persecutory conviction and grandiosity in each of the subtypes. Now DSMIV allows the simultaneous presence of more than one theme and it is sometimes legitimate to diagnose, let us say, jealousy and persecutory themes in the same patient. This makes no difference to the treatment approach so long as the diagnosis of delusional disorder is a firm one.

The presence of persecutory delusions naturally makes the patient extremely wary and guarded and it is not uncommon for people involved in his life to become incorporated in his delusional system (Cameron, 1959). This at times may include his physicians or, if he becomes litigious, members of the legal profession. (That aspect will be touched upon in the section on querulous or litigious paranoia, which is regarded as a variant of the persecutory subtype.) Delusional disorder sufferers are notoriously difficult to engage in treatment and persecutory ones especially so. A patient, low-key and nonjudgmental approach by the psychiatrist is necessary. Even so, the individual will often vent his anger on the latter and, on occasion, involve him or her in complaints or court situations. One cannot stress strongly enough the need to avoid any kind of confrontational situation, which is not easy when, for example, the psychiatrist may have had to sign committal papers for a patient's compulsory admission. Just as importantly, the psychiatrist should carefully document each transaction with the patient at the time it occurs so that it is possible later to refute any false accusations.

However, in other aspects, the treatment of the persecutory subtype is exactly as for the other subtypes and that will be discussed in full in Chapter 13.

An example of persecutory delusional disorder is described in Case No. 1 (see p.46).

'Querulous paranoia': a variation on delusional disorder, persecutory subtype

As Ungvari and Hollokoi (1993) point out, this variant of the persecutory subtype has a variety of names, including 'litigious paranoia', 'litigious delusional state', 'querulous paranoid state', 'querulent paranoia' and 'querulous paranoia' (querulent meaning complaining or peevish). They themselves add to that number by calling it querulant–litigious delusional disorder or QLDD. Rather illogically this author retains the term querulous paranoia, although one should perhaps have opted for querulous delusional disorder: however, it seems best not to make it seem another fully-fledged subtype of delusional disorder.

As always in the field of paranoia/delusional disorder, there is long-standing controversy about the concept and about the exact nature of the diagnosis involved. What we are discussing here are people who have a profound and persistent sense of having been wronged and who ceaselessly and endlessly seek redress, in some cases (hence the litigious element in the designation) seeking that redress through the legal system. Doubtless some of these individuals have suffered real grievances and have a strong sense of injustice which they are entitled to express, but it is inescapable that there are elements of psychiatric illness in at least a proportion of them and Rowlands (1988) describes cases in which paranoid personality disorder, paranoia or schizophrenia are involved. Naturally we shall be concentrating on those cases which fall into the paranoia category.

Kraepelin (1921) originally regarded querulous delusional states as the prototypical form of paranoia and included them in the group of persecutory paranoia cases. This is the stance adopted in the recent DSM and ICD series and the present author (Munro, 1982) has referred to it in these terms, but Astrup (1984) found only a proportion of his cases of querulent paranoia to have persecutory beliefs. So, Ungvari and Hollokoi (1993) suggest that they should formally be divided into two subgroups, those with and those without persecutory delusions: it is perhaps too soon to say whether this suggestion has merit, but it should be borne in mind.

Many patients with delusional disorder exhibit a peevish, complaintive quality but in querulous paranoia this is their most prominent feature, and their delusional system is one which is predominantly preoccupied with real or imagined wrongs and the need to obtain satisfaction for them. Litigious paranoia would appear to be that further subset in which the individual resorts incessantly to the legal system in order to pursue his unrequitable complaints.

As Rowlands (1988) points out, the overall group of those who persist in prolonged litigation for real or imagined injuries to themselves is small, and the subgroup who are mentally ill is smaller still. Within that subgroup are some who have delusional disorders, but they are seldom recognized as such in British or American courts. On the other hand, in Scandinavia and Germany there is an official diagnosis of querulent paranoia which the legal system can act upon, and reports occur in the legal and medical literatures on its phenomena and how it is handled. This is in contrast to the English language literature where descriptions of querulous and litigious paranoia are largely anecdotal, and are not reported in general psychiatric journals, so the average psychiatrist has little or no formal knowledge on the subject.

Winokur (1977) found that 5 out of 29 cases of delusional disorder showed litigious features or had persistent contacts with the law. There is a general consensus that litigious paranoia is not common but, as with other forms of delusional disorder, a relatively high functioning individual may be able to conceal the more psychotic aspects of his beliefs and Astrup (1984) reports that many remain in the community, sometimes still employed, although their delusions persist. Retterstøl (1975) claimed that litigious paranoia mostly occurred in males but d'Orban (1985) reports on a group of women in England and Wales sent to prison for contempt of court. These women tended to be older, one-third of them were immigrants and 37.5 percent had evidence of a psychiatric disorder. Of the mentally ill, some two-thirds had a 'paranoid disorder' which, since insufficient details are provided, might mean paranoid personality disorder, paranoid schizophrenia or delusional disorder: one must assume that some, at least, fell into this last category. d'Orban believed that diagnostic findings in the much larger number of male contempt offenders might be similar. An interesting finding, though backed with slight evidence, is that there appeared to be no excess of schizophrenia or mood disorder in the family histories of the paranoia patients, a finding which is consistent with the family history pattern in delusional disorder (see Chapter 2).

Goldstein (1987a), who has had much forensic psychiatric experience, describes three typical presentations of litigious paranoid states, which he describes as 'the hypercompetent defendant' (who knows the absolute letter of the law but nothing of the spirit); the 'paranoid party in a divorce proceeding', who is often consumed with jealousy and a sense of having been wronged and who may pursue vendettas, including some against judges; and the 'paranoid complaining witness' who incessantly pursues grievances. In each case, it may take a long time to recognize that such individuals are ill, unless an experienced psychiatrist becomes involved.

The subject would not be delusional disorder if there were no disagreements about the exact nature of diagnosis and of aetiology. Astrup (1984) adopted a Scandinavian stance when he described it as a 'psychogenic' psychosis (see Chapter 11) in which a key experience, such as a court case or dismissal from work, initiated the paranoid behaviour. McKenna (1984) saw the behaviour as being due to an overvalued idea rather than a delusion: one can only say that both nondelusional and delusional types of case very likely exist. Kolle (1931), Kretschmer (1927) and Schneider (1958) each emphasize abnormal, especially paranoid, personality factors as the basis of the abnormal beliefs and behaviour. Theorising apart, it is safe to say that a proportion of individuals who behave in an unreasonably litigious way will be mentally ill, and some of these will fulfil the criteria for delusional disorder.

Anyone who has dealt with querulous or litigious paranoids will appreciate the problems they pose, but for a vivid word-picture of such cases, one would recommend the reader to an article by Freckelton (1988), who writes as Manager of the Police Complaints Authority of the State of Victoria, Australia, and who clearly has first-hand experience in the field. He describes the 'querulant paranoid' as someone who has a compulsion to draw the attention of others to some wrong allegedly suffered. When such people become litigious nowadays they have, as Freckelton points out, limitless access to lawyers, courts, tribunals, review bodies, community justice mechanisms, and to the ombudsman. Legal aid, when available, gives them financial support and human rights initiatives have made the system much less resistant to them.

Freckelton notes that deluded litigants are often difficult to identify at first, but he provides a series of pointers for early recognition. According to him, the paranoid litigant shows:

(1) A determination to succeed against all the odds.
(2) A ready tendency to identify barriers as conspiracies.
(3) An endless crusading spirit to right a wrong (sometimes the original wrong being a real one).
(4) A driven quality, getting 'agonising' pleasure from pursuing the cause.
(5) Unsociability and quarrelsomeness.
(6) The 'scatter-gun' or 'blunderbuss' approach, saturating the field with multiple complaints.
(7) Suspiciousness in interviews.

These individuals readily fall out with their lawyers, refuse to pay their fees and threaten to complain to higher authority, which they often do. If thwarted they may take to unpleasant harassing tactics. In some cases they dismiss legal advice and conduct their own cases. They become expert at exploiting loopholes in rules of procedure and will pursue cases far beyond the bounds of reasonableness, sometimes losing sight of the original purpose of the whole process.

Unlike other writers, Freckelton says that litigious paranoia is not that rare. Legal manoeuvres to restrict these people exist but are often difficult to apply. His suggestion is that they should be identified as quickly as possible and treated humanely but firmly. That sounds like good advice, but anyone who has been caught up personally in a case of paranoia-driven litigation can attest to how difficult it is to counter an individual of this type or to see the process cut short.

Treatment and prognosis

The usual pessimism pervades the literature. Astrup (1984) says that treatment should be psychological but does not indicate how this should be initiated or how to get an insightless and unco-operative individual to comply. As with most traditional descriptions of paranoia, the general attitude is that treatment is unavailing and the condition unrelenting. However, on a more positive note, Ungvari and Hollokoi (1993) report on one case of litigious paranoia in an elderly man treated successfully on a maintenance dose of 2 mg of pimozide daily. The patient had had a delusional belief for almost 40 years but this was not recognized until he resorted to violent behaviour and was admitted to hospital. On medication his delusions gradually diminished, as typically happens in a good response in delusional disorder, and he was able to lead a normal existence for the first time in four decades.

Although that one report appears to stand alone at present, it seems likely that other patients with litigious or querulous paranoia could be equally helped. How to persuade these individuals to accept appropriate help or treatment is, of course, a wholly different question. There is also a realistic concern that over-ready willingness to diagnose paranoia in an excessively litigious person might lead to abuses of psychiatry, such as occurred in Russia in the past (Stålström, 1980). However, if some individuals who are mentally ill are being allowed to ride roughshod over the legal system and those on whom it impacts, it can surely be no bad thing at least to know the nature of their disorder and whether any kind of productive intervention is possible.

Case No. 9   Delusional disorder, persecutory subtype: with litigious features

A man of 82 who appeared to be in full possession of his intellectual faculties was referred for a psychiatric opinion. He was pleasant and co-operative, but totally unconvinced of the necessity of the interview. He showed a certain amount of humour, joking that his family thought he was 'crazy', but himself denying that he had any problems, psychological or otherwise.

Some 44 years previously, he and a business partner agreed to sever their relationship and wind up their joint company. Soon afterwards, the patient became convinced that the agreement had been drawn up to his severe disadvantage, and sought legal advice. Although his lawyer could not find any evidence to support his complaint, the patient insisted on going to court. He lost his case, but immediately re-cast his accusation in slightly different form and returned to court. He again lost, but in the ensuing 40 years or more, he had pressed his case innumerable times, always altering his plea slightly, and inevitably losing. He carried on even though his ex-partner died during the process; at the time of interview, he was still pursuing litigation.

He was a relatively wealthy man, but he had considerably neglected his business interests during much of this time, and members of his family largely took them over. His preoccupation led to his wife divorcing him, and his two sons becoming estranged from him. He was well aware of the havoc his fixation had produced, but insisted that he was right in his judgment about the original settlement and justified in pursing his litigation, although he had been told endless times that his case was hopeless. He knew that he had lost huge sums of money in legal fees and costs but was not deterred. 'The lawyers laugh at me, but they still take my money', he said, apparently seeing their willingness to take his money as evidence that they thought he did have a viable case.

He had been sent for a psychiatric interview at the insistence of family members who, it seemed, were more concerned about the loss of money from the family fortune caused by the patient's endless litigiousness, than they were about the patient himself. He showed some ideas of reference towards his family and towards the legal profession, but in general he was urbane, good-humoured and relatively well balanced except on the subject of his perpetual lawsuit. There, he had no insight whatsoever and had no recognition that the enormous cost in time and money was in any way unnecessary. He expressed regret about his family break-up but put the blame for it squarely on his wife and sons.

At the end of the assessment he politely declined a further interview and went off. During the following year, a local newspaper made a feature out of his 44-year-long legal saga and mentioned that he had recently gone to court once again on the same topic.

The dangerous paranoid patient

The great majority of psychiatric patients are not dangerous. So far as we can tell, this is also true of the great majority of delusional disorder patients (Goldstein, 1995), but we have so few reliable statistics in this area that we can only base such a statement on impression rather than on actual knowledge. Certainly there is a widespread apprehension about paranoid individuals who commit crimes, perhaps because there is a feeling that these people pursue their delusionally-driven aims to extreme ends and are not to be diverted by ordinary human considerations. And, of course, to most people paranoid means 'persecuted', which engenders a view of a deluded person who is set on revenge at all costs. The truth is that most deluded individuals suffer in isolation and do not act out their delusions but those who do certainly give cause for concern and even, at times, alarm.

Any illness associated with delusions may lead to criminal acts if the patient is sufficiently lacking in judgment and in normal levels of inhibition, but there are certain unique features in delusional disorder which make it especially dangerous. First, it is chronic and this allows the individual enormous time to brood on his beliefs. Secondly, the individual's intellectual ability, his thought form and his reasoning ability are relatively unimpaired. Thirdly, he often remains in society and continues to function, which in most people's minds betokens relative sanity.

So, when the delusional disorder patient develops his or her abnormal belief system, it may be based on incorrect premises and illogical thinking, but the delusions are often elaborate, ingenious and, at least superficially, highly plausible. Because the person remains in the community he can interweave imaginary beliefs with real events. If he is focusing his anger and resentfulness on other people, literally anything will fuel the flames of his suspicions and these become incorporated into the delusions (Kennedy, Kemp and Dyer, 1992). If judgment is becoming seriously affected and ordinary behavioural inhibitions are weakening, and especially if outbursts of anger are becoming more common, violent and possibly murderous behaviour may erupt. In general, it is males who are likely to behave most aggressively. Afterwards, the individual may feel and express regret but usually continues to believe that his action was totally justified.

It is not only the persecutory subtype of delusional disorder which gives rise to assault or murder. Violent cases involving erotomanic (Taylor, Mahendra and Gunn, 1983; Goldstein, 1987b) and jealousy (Shepherd, 1961; Mowat, 1966; Retterstøl, 1967) delusions are well documented, and some cases of sexual stalking are certainly related to delusional illnesses (Zona, Sharma and Lane, 1993).

For many years, the presence of delusions was one of the main legal criteria for determining insanity and the famous McNaghten rules of 1843 were the English legal system's attempt to define the relationship of delusion to crime (in this case murder). The House of Lords declared in essence that, 'to establish a defence on the ground of insanity, it must be clearly proved that at the time of committing the act, the party accused was labouring under such defect of reason, from disease of the mind, as not to know the nature and quality of the act he was doing, or if he did know it, that he did not know he was doing what was wrong' (quoted in Goldstein, 1995).

These rules have been modified over the years and, in their original form, are rarely applied in English law because they are generally agreed to be too narrow; it is impossible to regard an action as having taken place only because of a cognitive misapprehension since emotion, volition and capacity for behavioural control are obviously also important. Nevertheless, the spirit of the McNaghten rule still influences thinking in most of the judicial systems influenced by English Common Law.

It is ironic that the rules were devised to deal with a case of political assassination in which the murderer, David McNaghten, very likely suffered from a delusional disorder, and yet the law of insanity is particularly hard to apply to cases with this illness. Nowadays, the principal issue is whether or not the accused appreciated the rightfulness or wrongfulness of his action, and in many instances the delusional disorder sufferer is perfectly aware that, by societal standards, what he did was legally wrong. But that awareness lies within the normal and relatively undeteriorated aspects of his personality and cognition. Within his delusional system he fully believes that what he did was morally right and transcends any legal niceties. Not only does this put a judge and jury in a difficult decisional quandary, but their attitudes are bound to be affected by the accused's arrogance, self-justification, and lack of regret. In fact, the individual's ability to acknowledge the wrongness of his act in general terms, while refusing to accept that it was wrong for him specifically to commit it, may be seen as wilfulness or hypocrisy.

The odd result is, as Goldstein (1995) notes, that culpability may be determined by the content of the delusion. So, if the illegal act would have been appropriate had the circumstances been real, then the individual may be seen to have acted 'justifiably'. For example, if he felt threatened as a result of a delusion and acted – as he genuinely believed – in self defence, his degree of blame may be low; on the other hand, if he acted out of a desire for revenge, even if that desire is equally delusionally motivated, he may be regarded as warranting a higher degree of blame. There is a certain degree of illogic in this that almost matches the illogic of the individual's delusions.

The law is sometimes concerned with its own internal consistencies more than with any real appreciation of life as it actually exists. Insanity is seen as black and white and an illness like delusional disorder which contains both black and white is difficult for lawyers to understand. Although in no way an expert in forensic psychiatry, the present author has had experience of appearing in court to give evidence in cases of crime committed by persons with delusional disorder who had acted in response to their delusions. The outcome is a lottery: for example, in one such case there were three sittings under three different judges and, to this nonlegal mind, each of the judgments was contradictory to the others, even though the evidence and the issues were essentially the same on each occasion.

Much of the problem lies with the legal profession's preoccupation with its own rules, and its adherence to views on psychiatric illness which were discarded by psychiatrists many years ago. Our two professions speak different languages and have widely different credos. This was less of a problem when psychiatry's knowledge base was very static but now that it is rapidly becoming much more evidence-based and open to change, it is increasingly difficult for the lawyer and the psychiatrist to communicate meaningfully. In the case of delusional disorder there are additional problems in that we are still using especially unscientific concepts to define the illness and its symptoms, we have little systematic modern information on its features, and many psychiatrists remain unfamiliar with such up-to-date knowledge as exists. Little wonder that perplexity reigns when cases of delusional disorder are argued over in court.

These are important cases since, in many ways, they present issues in a seemingly clear-cut way that is not possible with more complex psychiatric disorders such as schizophrenia or major depression with delusions. A good deal of legislation on insanity continues to be based on major cases in which the accused had a delusional disorder (Goldstein, 1995, quotes the examples of Hinckley, who attempted to murder President Reagan, and Poddar, the deluded assailant in the Tarasoff case), and yet the advice which psychiatrists present to the court is too often quite erroneous. Again, perhaps the most important error to be perpetuated is that delusional disorder is largely untreatable, a view which is no longer tenable, as will be shown in Chapter 13.

Delusional disorder – grandiose subtype

Grandiosity or megalomania is described in several different psychiatric disorders, especially mania, delusional disorder, schizophrenia and cerebral syphilis (general paralysis of the insane). It is defined in DSMIV as follows:

An inflated appraisal of one's worth, power, knowledge, importance or identity. When extreme, grandiosity may be of delusional proportions.

In mania, the grandiosity is part of the elevated mood state, associated with euphoria, overactivity and lack of insight. In schizophrenia it may or may not be part of a euphoric presentation and in some patients there may be distinct incongruity between the expansive delusions and the relative thought poverty which exist side by side. In organic brain disorders, especially those affecting the pre-frontal lobes of the cerebrum, the manner is facile, the mood labile, and there are likely to be significant accompanying cognitive deficits. In all of these disorders, an element of irritability and suspiciousness often coexist with the grandiosity.

Delusional disorder, grandiose subtype, is the least well described of the subtypes of delusional disorder and the writer can only recall having seen two undoubted cases during a long career in psychiatry. Many individuals with other forms of delusional disorder show marked arrogance and hauteur, which seem to reflect a quality of exaggerated self-esteem, but cases predominantly characterized by grandiosity are rarely reported and the literature on the subject is very scanty.

Of course, one reason for the apparent rarity of the illness is its very nature. An individual who is extremely happy and even exalted, and who believes he is unbelievably rich and powerful, is perhaps the least likely of people to seek help from a psychiatrist. Because, as with other cases of delusional disorder, the patient remains sufficiently high-functioning in the community to maintain a quasi-normal existence, it is likely that his disorder will remain relatively unnoticed, particularly if it is channeled in some socially acceptable way – for example, belonging to a fringe religious group.

In the grandiose delusional disorder patient, as in other delusional disorder cases, there is the same quality of encapsulation of the delusional system, so that he or she is totally convinced of the false beliefs while otherwise still living in an everyday world. For some people this situation may continue indefinitely but, for others, one of two things may happen. Either they may withdraw further and further into their fantasy world and cease to care for themselves adequately, or they may begin to act out their delusions, spending nonexistent money, behaving outrageously or, as with the hero of Pirandello's play, *Henry IV*, bending reality to fit his abnormal beliefs.

It seems possible, or even likely, that some individuals with grandiose beliefs can adopt a lifestyle which accommodates and sanctions their delusions and their behaviour. The most obvious way in which this can occur is, as mentioned, by participation in the kind of extreme apocalyptic religious group which allows the person to share and even propagate his strange beliefs. The infamous Jonestown massacre (Weightman, 1984), in which nearly 1000 people died, would appear to have resulted from a combination of a charismatic but deluded leader, the Reverend Bob Jones, a small group of equally deluded individuals, another group of people with a version of *folie à deux* and, lastly, a large number of victims. The Waco incident (Reavis, 1995) seems to have similar connotations. Comparable scenarios appear to occur in some of the ultra-extreme paramilitary groups which have become notorious in the United States, where grandiose and persecutory delusions mingle and prophecies of Armageddon thrive (Myers, 1988). A re-reading of the lives of the Nazi leaders, especially Hitler (Toland, 1984) and Hess (Padfield, 1995), leads this author to believe at least in the possibility that some of these men could have been charismatic paranoiacs.

The megalomania of delusional disorder is a sustained phenomenon since the illness, like any delusional disorder, is likely to be chronic. It may apparently appear gradually or suddenly, affect both sexes, and occur at any age. As indicated, it may or may not be acted out. Its origin is obscure. Freud proposed that it is a development of narcissism – self-regard which becomes increasingly pathological in degree as the result of the investment of the self with libido which is usually invested in external objects (Swanson, Bohnert and Smith, 1970). This seems a very pale explanation when one is faced with the intensity of the actual phenomenon and the abnormality of its beliefs. A related theory is that grandiosity may represent a prolongation of the feelings of omnipotence said to occur in the young child, which is plausible but not particularly helpful either.

A common theory of grandiosity is that it is secondary to, or a flight from, feelings of worthlessness. This view would be easier to sustain in a mood disorder setting, but in delusional disorder so many patients show minor forms of grandiosity – especially a curt, condescending manner and a conviction of superior knowledge – that it seems much more likely to be a primary feature. It is generally believed that grandiosity represents a particularly severe degree of psychopathology. This may be so, but the well organised and stable grandiose delusional system is so often associated with unassailable complacency that it is impossible to gain any foothold for treatment. This may not represent additional severity, but rather an understandable reluctance of the patient to abandon his highly pleasurable beliefs.

Sometimes, the grandiosity of delusional disorder is not unalloyed, and it may be associated with anger and suspicion, and the world is seen as a hostile place. This seems a particularly dangerous combination and Goldstein (1995) gives graphic descriptions of deluded individuals who have a sense of their own uniqueness and infallibility and become highly dangerous members of society.

An interesting element in grandiosity is that of *centrality* (Swanson, Bohnert and Smith, 1970). Here, the individual feels that he is the centre of attention all the time. Highly unusual and improbable things happen to him, yet he does not question these. Why, for example, should an obscure and inoffensive Englishman be singled out by the Irish Republican Army as someone who must be assassinated, or a very ordinary New Yorker feel that he is being constantly shadowed by the FBI? A patient who believes that he is being spied upon will never see it as unlikely that many millions of pounds or dollars would have to be spent to maintain this surveillance. Centrality is often associated with ideas of reference and persecution but can also be characterized by feelings of bliss if the delusion is an exalted or religious one.

Presumably the treatment of delusional disorder, grandiose subtype, is the same as for other subtypes but there appears to be no evidence for this, apart from one communication the present author obtained from a colleague (Adelman, 1984, personal communication), who treated such a patient with pimozide and reported a successful outcome with this. Prior to treatment it is essential that a careful mental examination be carried out and a thorough differential diagnosis be performed.

Case No. 10   Delusional disorder, grandiose subtype

A respectable, middle-class woman of 53, divorced and living alone, was required to have a psychiatric assessment after being charged with creating a disturbance. She had wakened a quiet suburb late at night by ringing a handbell and shouting slogans. Her rationale was that the developer of the neighbourhood property was Muslim and that this was therefore not a fit place for Christian people to live in. She was unperturbed at being arrested, charged or referred for interview, saying that this had happened to her before and that it gave her more opportunity to spread her message 'to all the peoples'.

She answered questions politely. She said she was employed in a civil service post (at a relatively low level, it was determined) and lived a very circumscribed life. Her only interest outside work was in the 'philosophy of religion' and she belonged to several fringe groups and societies dealing with this. From time to time she felt the urge to demonstrate her beliefs publicly and planned beforehand how to create the most noticeable effect.

The patient appeared intelligent and, on first contact, seemed relatively normal. However, as soon as her pet subject was touched upon, her whole manner changed. She became possessed, elated, grandiose and at times derisory. There was no flight of ideas but marked pressure of speech was present, and she harangued the interviewer with her credo, which sounded superficially understandable but finally appeared to make no sense. When gently interrupted and brought on to a neutral topic, she quickly settled down and talked logically and reasonably. She appeared to enjoy good physical health and, so far as could be determined, had thought and behaved like this all her adult life.

At the end of the interview she declined any help, and gave the interviewer several tracts written by herself which she said would clear up any uncertainties which might have arisen in the course of the conversation. She said that she had been commended by many people for her brilliant writing style which was, in fact, opaque and extremely vague. She was not seen again by the interviewer.

References

Astrup C. (1984). Querulent paranoia: a follow-up. *Neuropsychobiology* **11**: 149–154.

Cameron, N. 1959 The paranoid pseudocommunity revisited. *Am. J. Sociol.* **65**: 57–61.

Diagnostic and Statistical Manual of Mental Disorders, 4th edn. (DSMIV) (1994). Washington, DC: American Psychiatric Association.

Freckelton, I. (1988). Querulent paranoia and the vexatious complainant. *Int. J. Law Psychiat.* **11**: 127–143.

Goldstein, R.L. (1987a). Litigious paranoids and the legal system: the role of the forensic psychiatrist. *J. Forens. Sci. JFSCA* **32**: 1009–1115.

Goldstein, R.L. (1987b). More forensic romances: de Clérambault's syndrome in men. *Bull. Am. Acad. Psychiat. Law* **15**: 267–274.
Goldstein, R.L. (1995). Paranoids in the legal system: the litigious paranoid and the paranoid criminal. *Psychiat. Clin. N. Am.* **18**: 303–315.
International Statistical Classification of Diseases, 10th edn. (ICD10) (1992–3). Geneva: World Health Association.
Kennedy, H.G., Kemp, L.I. and Dyer, D.E. (1992). Fear and anger in delusional (paranoid) disorder: the association with violence. *Br. J. Psychiat.* **160**: 488–492.
Kolle, K. (1931). Über Querulanten. *Arch. Psychiat. Nervenkrankh.* **95**: 24–100.
Kraepelin, E. (1921). *Manic-depressive Insanity and Paranoia*. Transl. R.M. Barclay (1976). New York: Arno Press.
Kretschmer, E. (1927). *Der sensitive Beziehungswahn*, 2nd edn. Berlin: Springer.
McKenna, P.J. (1984). Disorders with overvalued ideas. *Br. J. Psychiat.* **145**: 579–585.
Mowat, R.R. (1966). *Morbid Jealousy and Murder*. London: Tavistock Publications.
Munro, A. (1982). Paranoia revisited. *Br. J. Psychiat.* **141**: 344–349.
Myers, P.L. (1988). Paranoid pseudocommunity beliefs in a sect milieu. *Soc. Psychiat. Psychiatr. Epidemiol.* **23**: 252–255.
d'Orban, P.T. (1985). Psychiatric aspects of contempt of court among women. *Psycholog. Med.* **15**: 597–607.
Padfield, P. (1995). *Hess: The Führer's Disciple*. London: MacMillan.
Reavis, D.J. (1995). *Ashes of Waco: An Investigation*. New York: Simon and Shuster.
Retterstøl, N. (1975). *The Labyrinths of the Mind*. Oslo: Universitetsforlaget.
Retterstøl, N. (1967). Jealousy–paranoiac psychoses. *Acta Psychiat. Scand.* **43**: 75–107.
Rowlands, M.W.D. (1988). Psychiatric and legal aspects of persistent litigation. *Br. J. Psychiat.* **153**: 317–323.
Schneider, K. (1958). *Psychopathic Personalities*, transl. M.W. Hamilton, London: Cassell.
Shepherd, M. (1961). Morbid jealousy: some clinical and social aspects of a psychiatric syndrome. *J. Ment. Sci.* **107**: 687–753.
Stålström, O.W. (1980). Querulous paranoia: diagnosis and dissent. *Aust. N. Z. J. Psychiat.* **14**: 145–150.
Swanson, D.W., Bohnert, P.J. and Smith, J.A. (1970). *The Paranoid*. Boston: Little, Brown and Co.
Taylor, P., Mahendra, B. and Gunn, J. (1983). Erotomania in males. *Psycholog. Med.* **13**: 645–650.
Toland, J. (1984). *Adolf Hitler*. New York: Ballantine Books.
Ungvari, G.S. and Hollokoi, R.I.M. (1993). Successful treatment of litigious paranoia with pimozide. *Can. J. Psychiat.* **38**: 4–8.
Weightman, J.M. (1984). *Making Sense of the Jonestown Suicides: Sociological History of Peoples Temple*. Lewiston, NY: Edwin Mellen Press.
Winokur, G. (1977). Delusional disorder (paranoia). *Comp. Psychiat.* **18**: 511–521.
Zona, M.A., Sharma, K.K. and Lane, J. (1993). A comparative study of erotomanic and obsessional subjects in a forensic sample. *J. Forens. Sci., JFSCA* **38**: 894–903.

Part III

'Paranoid spectrum' illnesses which should be included in the category of delusional disorder

... in wand'ring mazes lost.
John Milton (1608–1674)

Psychiatrists frequently talk about 'schizophrenic spectrum' or 'depressive spectrum' disorders, implying a group of illnesses with significant phenomenological or psychopathological relationships to each other. Illnesses in the spectrum need not themselves be schizophrenia or major mood disorder, but may well be cognates or precursors.

Delusional disorder, as at present featured in ICD10 and DSMIV, is both an illness and a category, since only one delusional disorder is described – an updated version of the venerable paranoia. But when paranoia was a well-accepted diagnosis in the late nineteenth and early twentieth centuries, it was frequently seen as a member of a group of paranoid illnesses and, in Chapter 7, the concept of a 'paranoid spectrum' is discussed. In addition to paranoia, paraphrenia and paranoid schizophrenia were members of that grouping.

Nowadays, paraphrenia is neglected and paranoid schizophrenia, although clearly distinct in many ways from the rest of schizophrenia, is included with the latter. In addition we have other disorders hovering uncertainly in the background, including 'late' paraphrenia (a controversial entity) and schizophrenia of late onset, which is increasingly being recognized; also, there is the group of illnesses which make up the delusional misidentification syndromes, which has little or no official provenance at all.

This writer has repeatedly made the case that the revival of paranoia/delusional disorder in DSMIIIR was a job only half done. At the very least paraphrenia should also have been recognized and included in the category. In addition, there is a case – and some very attractive advantages could accrue from it – for placing most or all of the individual conditions described in Part III under the heading of delusional disorder. This is not to say that they are the same as paranoia/delusional disorder but to suggest that they belong on a continuum with it.

Finally, we look at *folie à deux*, not so much to say that it is a delusional disorder but to stress that it is a phenomenon related to all illnesses with delusions. It is a good deal less rare than usually thought and Chapter 10 suggests a number of practical reasons why it should never be overlooked.

7
Paraphrenia and paranoid schizophrenia

Paraphrenia

Introduction

Paraphrenia was introduced as a distinct condition by Emil Kraepelin (1921) early in the twentieth century and he described it as a functional psychotic disorder which was separate from both schizophrenia and paranoia. Paraphrenia suffered a similar fate to paranoia as the definition of schizophrenia later began to widen, and eventually most cases were probably diagnosed as paranoid schizophrenia or, as now seems to be becoming more common, schizoaffective disorder. Paranoia, as we have seen, has re-emerged since DSMIIIR (1987) in recent years as a diagnosis in its own right, although re-named delusional disorder. Paraphrenia is currently excluded from the principal diagnostic classificatory systems, but still has a shadowy existence on the edge of our psychiatric nosology.

This chapter aims to demonstrate that paraphrenia is at the very least a sub-category of psychiatric illness whose diagnosis is of practical value, and that it may possibly even be a separate diagnostic entity. Of late, psychiatrists appear to have become increasingly unwilling to diagnose schizophrenia when there are significantly atypical features present but, as will be noted, there is often no satisfactory alternative diagnostic category for cases like this. In fact, some of these 'atypical' patients' illnesses accord well with the description of paraphrenia, particularly when the latter is modified in terms of modern concepts and practices (see later).

Diagnostic difficulties in psychiatry: in general and in particular

In the majority of psychiatric disorders we still utilize relatively little technology in making a diagnosis and rely instead on history-taking and careful observation. Although research on the central nervous system is continually demonstrating a growing number of increasingly subtle brain abnormalities and is beginning to link these to abnormal mental phenomena, clinical applications of these methodologies remain disappointingly slow.

Psychiatry now possesses a range of powerful treatments which can be applied to illnesses whose characteristics are still only imperfectly understood. The moment a treatment is started, the appearance and the course of the illness are altered – we hope beneficially, although sometimes the opposite occurs. It is therefore rarely possible nowadays to observe the unmodified natural history of a psychiatric disorder, except in patients who refuse treatment. No one wishes to return to the therapeutic nihilism of earlier times, but our modern therapies have taken away the opportunity to follow the evolution of psychiatric disorders. This means that we have to make most of our diagnoses on a very limited, cross-sectional basis. Undoubtedly technology will catch up as in other specialties and allow more objective assessments to be made, but in the meantime the psychiatrist often has to apply very specific treatments to cases whose diagnoses are, to say the least, tentative.

As well as this, an important variable in diagnosis is the credo to which each psychiatrist adheres. It is only quite recently that we have begun to adopt widely acceptable definitions of the illnesses in our specialty and a standardised terminology with which to describe them. An example of the past from which we are beginning to dissociate ourselves is the confusion which became obvious in the 1950s or thereabouts regarding the diagnosis of schizophrenia in the United Kingdom and the United States. It took a carefully co-ordinated study to show that the illness was not twice as common in America as in Britain as appeared in the statistics, but was instead grossly over-diagnosed in the former country because of particular philosophical and diagnostic practices there (Gurland and colleagues, 1970).

For many years it has been customary to refer to 'the schizophrenias' (Harris and Jeste, 1988), because the category so obviously contains a number of illnesses with certain common resemblances. As time passes, this impression of heterogeneity is increasingly confirmed but yet, in our clinical work, we go on diagnosing schizophrenia as though it were an entity, accepting poorly validated clinical subtypes such as the disorganised, the paranoid, and so on, and having to utilize large residual categories when the features of the individual case are indeterminate. Also, we have to accept the varying responses to identical treatments in different patients which must, we assume, reflect considerable variations in the underlying pathologies.

There is no question that schizophrenia is diagnosed much more carefully now than in the past, but it is impossible to be satisfied with our diagnostic practices with regard to the schizophrenic spectrum of disorders. It seems clear that there will be no one answer in the future for schizophrenia; the likelihood is that more and more subgroups with coherent features and specific treatment responses will be identified and removed from the overall category until a small core group, or nothing at all, is left. In the present chapter, paraphrenia is put forward as one of these subgroups with a recommendation that it be separated from schizophrenia.

Can paraphrenia be distinguished from schizophrenia?

A criterion which has sometimes been used to subclassify schizophrenia is whether cases are 'good outcome' or 'poor outcome'. In the past, when no worthwhile treatments were available, most cases of schizophrenia-like illness had a bad prognosis unless one included patients whose diagnosis of schizophrenia was, at best, dubious. Modern treatment has radically changed the picture and, in recent years, we have been watching undoubted cases of failed-treatment schizophrenia change from a bad prognosis to a reasonably good prognosis with the use of new atypical neuroleptics.

All psychiatrists know of cases which are similar to schizophrenia but whose symptoms are less florid and whose prognosis seems to be less dire. Even now, we are often forced to give these a relatively meaningless label such as 'atypical psychosis' (atypical of what?) or 'psychotic disorder NOS'. Increasingly, patients like this are being called 'schizoaffective disorder' which, if one looks at its criteria, is to a great extent another residual category. None of these pseudo-diagnoses is a satisfactory resort since they all of necessity lump together disparate, leftover cases. One of these leftovers, this author would aver, is paraphrenia, no longer recognized in the DSM or ICD series although, in this author's view, it has considerable clinical validity.

Paraphrenia: the background

In Chapter 1 the apparent demise and eventual reappearance of paranoia (now named delusional disorder) was described. The equally convoluted history of paraphrenia was also mentioned, but as yet it has failed to gain official rehabilitation. Emil Kraepelin (1921), as we saw, described both illnesses in detail, carefully distinguishing paranoia from dementia praecox (which Bleuler (1950) subsequently renamed schizophrenia), and in the eighth edition of Kraepelin's textbook (1909–1913) we see the introduction of the separate category of paraphrenia (a term originally devised by Kahlbaum in 1863).

Since Kraepelin's day, paraphrenia has continued to be diagnosed by some psychiatrists, often on idiosyncratic criteria, but in modern times the majority neither use the term nor view the condition as separate. Kraepelin's original definition was of a disorder similar to paranoid schizophrenia, with fantastic delusions and hallucinations, but having relatively slight thought disorder and much better affective preservation. Compared with schizophrenia there was less personality deterioration and volition was less impaired. In general, paraphrenic patients showed less disturbance of behaviour and even when their delusions were severe their manner appeared fairly reasonable. Their ability to communicate with others and to demonstrate rapport and affective warmth remained good.

Descriptions of paraphrenia in the literature

These will only be lightly touched upon here. What emerges as one pursues the literature chronologically is an early enthusiasm for Kraepelin's description, then an increasingly critical attitude, and thereafter a long period of neglect which continues to the present day. As a result of this neglect, the concept has failed to develop in line with modern nosological thought.

Kraepelin's original description of paraphrenia is reasonably convincing, so why is it then that a respected authority with a second-to-none track record in the description of mental illnesses could recognize paraphrenia as a separate illness, yet not persuade his successors of its legitimacy?

There is no simple answer in the literature. Some authors have clearly supported the concept, as when Anderson and Trethowan (1973) described paraphrenia as being less deteriorative than schizophrenia while not having the full characteristics of paranoia, and when Arieti (1955) noted that there was minimal personality destruction in paraphrenia although the illness itself was often deteriorative. Curran and Partridge (1969) stressed a factor which is often regarded as of key importance in diagnosis when they said that, in paraphrenia, emotional rapport remained 'strikingly' good, and Leonhard (1960) also emphasized the presence of strong affect in paraphrenia, although he did not separate it clearly from schizophrenia.

The preservation of good affective features in a schizophrenia-like illness has consistently been one of the most important diagnostic elements in paraphrenia. To illustrate its significance the following two case examples are presented.

Case No. 11   Paraphrenia in a middle-aged man

The patient is a 45-year-old married man who has been re-admitted to his local psychiatric hospital seven times in the past 17 years. The admissions are all fairly similar. After a varying period of relative well-being at home on medication, he stops taking his neuroleptic and over the next several weeks becomes deluded, hallucinated, and very disorganised in his behaviour. His delusions are multiple but the predominant one is usually that the local police are after him for a petty crime he committed as a teenager. He gets very angry at times and on more than one occasion has attacked a policeman. When psychotic he has no insight and his thinking is markedly disorganised.

Despite the severity of these episodes, when admitted to hospital he is pleasant to staff, shows very good emotional range with appropriate affect, and has a warm, empathic manner which makes him a favourite on the ward. When neuroleptic treatment is re-started he settles down over a period of two to three weeks and is discharged home. His wife and family are always glad to see him return and his employer is keen to have him start work as soon as possible. He has a number of hobbies when he is well. His longest period of good health was four years and his relapses always seem to be due to his stopping his medication.

Between episodes he is cheerful, a hard worker, and a popular community member. At interview when he is well he shows some looseness of associations and slight concreteness of thinking and there are occasional minor lapses of judgment. Otherwise his personality is remarkably well preserved.

For a considerable time he was diagnosed either as having paranoid schizophrenia or a schizoaffective disorder. He is now diagnosed as having paraphrenia.

Case No. 12   Paraphrenia in an older female

The patient is a 60-year-old clerical worker, married for more than 30 years and with three adult sons. Her childhood and early adult life were unremarkable and there is no history of psychiatric illness in her immediate family. She says that her marriage has always been dysfunctional because of her husband's alcoholism and emotional abuse. She left him two years ago and divorce proceedings are in progress. She appears to be effective in her daily work and has no severe money worries.

She was admitted to hospital in a very distressed state, saying that her husband was systematically persecuting her. In the past two months this had become constant and during the past two to three weeks, 'someone' had been gaining access to her apartment. She found the lock had been changed, papers had been scattered or stolen and handprints had been left on her walls. She was afraid to go to sleep and had had to give up work ten days ago. In the past week she had heard her husband's voice 'as though he could put his thoughts into my head' but denied that her apartment was 'bugged'. She believed all of this persecution was to enable her husband to get an unfair advantage over her in the divorce proceedings.

This is the fourth similar episode she has had in 12 years. She visits a psychiatrist who prescribes a neuroleptic drug which she does not mind taking and which, she agrees, helps her symptoms. However, from time to time she stops the medication for no apparent reason and gradually relapses. She now says she realises this is foolish of her.

Even when very distressed she is a personable woman, well groomed and looking younger than her actual age. Her story is convincing, her emotion genuinely appropriate and her insight seemingly good. She is happy to resume her medication and within several days is calm and asking if she can pay a visit to her apartment. Affect is warm, rapport is good and she has a pleasant sense of humour. On the other hand, she seems oddly oblivious of the fact that she felt so persecuted on admission and does not try to explain what was happening. Ten days after admission she says she is ready to return home and is looking forward to celebrating Christmas with her sons. She is quite willing to resume her visits to the psychiatrist.

It is interesting that, in contrast to the detailed descriptions of the content of delusions in paranoia/delusional disorder, the literature says almost nothing about the nature of the delusions which are prominent in paraphrenia. Sullivan (1962) mentions persecutory delusions and Lewis (1970) refers to an erotic content in some patients, but neither reference is convincingly attributed. In line with the prevailing contradictoriness in this literature, we find on the one hand a reference to unremitting systematized delusions and hallucinations in one source (Black, Yates and Andreasen, 1988), and to a lack of that quasi-logical systematisation of the delusions which is typical of paranoia in another (Kolb, 1973).

Brink and colleagues (1979) stated that patients suffering from paraphrenia retain reality testing except for the persistent delusion, but they may be describing paranoia/delusional disorder instead. Merskey (1980) cited patients with 'paranoid states or psychoses' whose illness commenced after the age of 35 and who did not evince the typical general deterioration of schizophrenia, and his description could be construed as referring to paraphrenia. Lewis (1970) suggested that paraphrenia was milder than schizophrenia and had a later onset, but Bleuler underlined paraphrenia's chronic, unremitting quality until, that is, he changed his mind and decided that paraphrenia was not separate from schizophrenia after all.

The DSMIII (1980) section on paranoid disorders confused paranoia and paraphrenia in its section on 'paranoia'. Subsequently DSMIIIR (1987) and DSMIV (1994) got their descriptions of paranoia/delusional disorder substantially right, but both completely excluded paraphrenia; ICD9 (1978) had an inaccurate definition of paraphrenia but the disorder has totally vanished from ICD10 (1992–1993).

As was described in Chapter 1, Mayer's study in 1921 seems to have greatly dampened enthusiasm for paraphrenia since he found that more than half of Kraepelin's 78 patients diagnosed as paraphrenic later developed schizophrenia. However, like Kolle's (1931) work on the follow-up of paranoia (see p.16), Mayer and other succeeding authors failed to emphasize that the remaining cases remained distinctively paraphrenic. Since Mayer's study, many psychiatrists have ignored paraphrenia or, at most, have regarded it putatively as a sub-variety of paranoid schizophrenia. Both Henderson and Batchelor (1962) and Fish (1964) advocated dropping it altogether and Lewis (1970) was unenthusiastic about its retention, saying that Kraepelin's paraphrenics could have been labelled 'paranoid' (by which he appears to mean 'suffering from paranoia') if they had only lacked hallucinations. Lewis fails to recognize that the delusions of paraphrenia lack the essential encapsulated quality typical of those in paranoia/delusional disorder.

Leigh and colleagues (1977) simply stated that paraphrenia is 'schizophrenia arising for the first time after the age of 60 years', which is untrue but is a convenient way to diagnose first-time schizophrenia in the elderly without getting into an ideological argument. Kraepelin's term 'dementia praecox' had emphasized the 'precocious' onset of schizophrenia but he himself accepted that some cases developed in later life. Despite this, most authorities came to believe that schizophrenia occurred for the first time no later than middle age. This became virtually a tenet of faith and so cases arising in the 60s or later, often with relatively good personality preservation, had to be found another name and, for some psychiatrists, the label of paraphrenia was one of these.

Now we are much more prepared to diagnose first-onset schizophrenia in older patients, although some psychiatrists are not wholly comfortable about this. The concepts of old age schizophrenia and late paraphrenia will be discussed later (see Chapter 8).

In reading the literature one gains the strong impression that the great majority of psychiatrists, whether they opt for paraphrenia or against it, are still quite unfamiliar with the distinctions between individual members of the delusional disorder group and often cannot separate these conceptually from schizophrenia. Since Mayer's study of 1921 there have been few or no original investigations on paraphrenia with the exception of studies on late paraphrenia which, as we shall see, is not quite the same thing. When paraphrenia was dropped from DSMIIIR (1987), Williams (1987) officially replied to an enquiry about its absence as follows:

Some argue that such a clinical picture distinguishes a unique syndrome and should be differentiated from schizophrenia. However, the general consensus among experts in the area is that it is premature to consider such a syndrome to be a separate disorder. Therefore, until further research proves or disproves its validity, it will still be diagnosed as schizophrenia.

That was in 1987 and paranoia remains a pariah. It is puzzling to know who these 'experts' are, whom Williams refers to, who excluded paraphrenia from DSMIIIR and DSMIV, since there is virtually no modern-day expertise or scholarly work on the subject. Yet, oddly, there are quite a few psychiatrists who continue to employ the term 'paraphrenia' in their clinical work, even if not always sure of its precise meaning.

What if paraphrenia does exist and is being diagnosed as schizophrenia (Williams, 1987), psychotic disorder NOS, or as schizoaffective disorder?

Does this really matter? The writer suggests it does because, if it is lumped in with a variety of other illnesses, it will be impossible to study in isolation. The present author and two colleagues, Drs A. Ravindran and L. Yatham, probably are as close to experts on paraphrenia as exist nowadays, and we have recently carried out an investigation in which we attempted to identify cases of paraphrenia, using criteria which will be detailed later in the present chapter. Our results are as yet unpublished but we believe that it is indeed possible to diagnose paraphrenia and distinguish it from other similar disorders (Ravindran and Yatham, personal communication, 1997). Given similar criteria it would not be difficult for other psychiatrists to follow our example.

The paranoid spectrum: a venerable concept (Munro, 1982)

For many years there has been a persistent theory that paranoia and paranoid schizophrenia represent opposite ends of a continuum of psychotic disorders in which delusions are a prominent feature. Figure 7.1 displays a schema showing paranoia/delusional disorder to the left, paranoid schizophrenia to the right and paraphrenia in the middle. 'Cluster A' personality disorders (DSMIV) are provisionally linked to the 'paranoia' end of the spectrum but lie outside it. Paranoid schizophrenia is included in the continuum because it has features in common with delusional disorders, but other forms of schizophrenia remain separate. Dementia is also shown to the right of the spectrum since a minority of paranoid spectrum cases have an underlying organic aetiology which eventually expresses itself as dementia. The misidentification disorders, which appear to have some features in common with the delusional disorders, but currently have no identified locus in standard diagnostic systems, are tentatively shown in association with paranoia/delusional disorder.

A proportion of individuals with severe forms of cluster A personality disorder eventually develop psychotic features (Jette and Winnett, 1987; Roth, 1955): when this occurs, there is some evidence that they are especially liable to develop a delusional disorder.

Approximately 10 per cent of patients with paranoia/delusional disorder or paraphrenia will show a 'shift to the right', deteriorating to schizophrenia or (especially in some older individuals) to dementia (Black, Yates and Andreasen, 1988). However, the majority of cases of delusional disorder and paraphrenia appear to remain diagnostically stable over long periods: despite this, many of them continue to be mistaken as schizophrenic or even mood disorder illnesses.

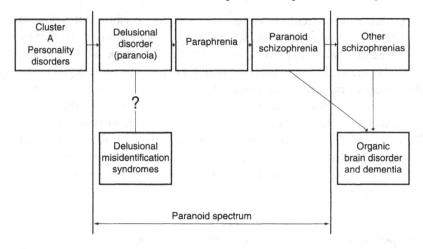

Fig. 7.1 The paranoid spectrum

Several reports have suggested that, as one moves from right to left on the spectrum, a family history of schizophrenia becomes progressively less common, which seems to indicate that the delusional disorders are relatively unrelated to schizophrenia genetically (Munro, 1982; Watt, 1985). Delusional disorder itself shows no more tendency to a family history of schizophrenia than among members of the general public.

Although paranoid schizophrenia is conventionally grouped with the other clinical forms of schizophrenia, there are cogent arguments for regarding it as separate and even for including it in the paranoid spectrum. Kraepelin is once more the authority most responsible for our present-day concepts on paranoid schizophrenia, a category which has proved much less controversial than paranoia or paraphrenia. He regarded it as a sub-category of dementia praecox but, as noted previously (see p.9), also included it in his group of paranoid disorders. Rather than indulging in pointless argument about where paranoid schizophrenia actually lies in some hypothesised diagnostic scheme, it is perhaps best to acknowledge its relative separateness from other forms of schizophrenia or from delusional disorder, while recognising that it has features in common with both of these illnesses.

Some mention of paranoid schizophrenia will be made later (see pp.162–165). In the meantime, as noted, some would argue that paraphrenia is, at most, a sub-set of paranoid schizophrenia. This may be true but, as will be shown, there are features that separate it from the latter and make it a potentially viable diagnosis in its own right. Also, there is a considerable gap in the paranoid spectrum between the constructs of delusional disorder and paranoid schizophrenia. There are cases which fall into that gap and paraphrenia appears to be a satisfactory diagnostic description for at least some of these.

A description of paraphrenia

The earlier part of this chapter has attempted to deal with some of the many ambiguities which surround paraphrenia: now we shall attempt to define and describe it. Because of the virtual absence of modern descriptions, the present author (Munro, 1991) devised a description, utilising modern terminology, a DSM-style format and the limited available data. As already mentioned, with Drs Ravindran and Yatham's co-operation, and using the under-noted criteria, a small case-finding study has been carried out whose results are currently being analysed. From this, we can say with some confidence that we were able to recognize cases of paraphrenia in two separate inpatient psychiatric settings. Our experiences give this writer considerable confidence in providing the following account of the illness.

Proposed diagnostic criteria for paraphrenia (Munro, 1991)

Paraphrenia is a distinct delusional disorder which must have been present for at least six months and is characterized by:

(1) Preoccupation with one or more semi-systematized delusions, often accompanied by auditory hallucinations. These delusions are not encapsulated from the rest of the personality.
(2) The affect remaining notably well preserved and relatively appropriate. Even when severely disturbed the patient shows an ability for rapport with others and considerable affective warmth which is not typical of any form of schizophrenia.
(3) None of the following: intellectual deterioration, visual hallucinations, incoherence, marked loosening of associations, flat or grossly inappropriate affect, grossly disorganised behaviour.
(4) Understandability of disturbed behaviour as being related to the content of the patient's delusions and hallucinations.
(5) The absence of significant organic brain disorder and, at most, only partial agreement with criterion A for schizophrenia in DSMIV.

Associated features

In general, the personality is better retained than in schizophrenia and patients remain relatively higher functioning (especially if they accept treatment). They may be able to conceal their delusional beliefs and behave outwardly in a relatively normal way, at least for a time. However, potential distress and agitation are almost invariably present, partly because some degree of insight is often retained. As the delusions grow stronger and judgment deteriorates, irrational behaviour becomes more obvious. The patient may accuse others of intimidation, make complaints to the authorities, or sometimes show aggression to imagined persecutors. At first, the apparent justifications for such actions may be fairly convincing and may mislead the observer.

Age of onset

Traditionally it is believed that the illness begins predominantly in middle or old age, even appearing for the first time in extreme old age. In fact, the author and his colleagues, A. Ravindran and L. Yatham, have found apparently typical cases among individuals as young as in their 20s, and in others as high as in their 80s.

Course and prognosis

Once established, it is a chronic illness, ameliorated but not cured by treatment. It tends to cause the patient to become withdrawn and isolated, which exacerbates the social and behavioural deterioration, thereby causing further symptoms. Unfortunately, a proportion of patients, prompted by their delusional beliefs, are noncompliant with treatment, which prolongs the acute phase, sometimes indefinitely. Not uncommonly, a pattern asserts itself of improvement in hospital followed by relapse in the community due to failure to take medication. In older patients who eventually become permanently institutionalised and whose treatment can be more closely supervised, improvement seems to be well maintained unless, for example, dementia supervenes. Because no population figures for the frequency of paraphrenia are available and because no research on the entity has been carried out for such a long time, we have no idea of the relative commonness of compliance versus noncompliance in a treated population, but noncompliance does seem to occur with more than random frequency.

Frequency of paraphrenia

Fenton, McGlashan and Heinssen (1988) were studying a series of patients who had been diagnosed as suffering from schizophrenia, using both DSMIII and DSMIIIR criteria. They found that approximately 10 per cent of those who were regarded as schizophrenic utilising DSMIII had to be excluded from the diagnosis when the stricter DSMIIIR criteria were applied. They noted that many of the excluded cases had symptoms of a delusional (paranoid) type, but had to be labelled as atypical psychoses because their delusions lacked the encapsulated quality of DSMIIIR delusional disorder.

It seems possible that many of the excluded cases could be seen as lying on the paranoid spectrum between delusional disorder and paranoid schizophrenia, i.e. in the position said to be occupied by paraphrenia (Munro, 1989). If that is so, then the frequency of paraphrenia in an inpatient psychiatric population could be provisionally estimated as being about one-tenth that of schizophrenia.

In 1982, Kendler found that patients with delusional disorders (not restricted to the DSMIIIR definition which had not then been devised) made up between 1 and 4 per cent of psychiatric admissions and between 2 and 7 per cent of functional psychoses. As shown in Chapter 2, an extrapolation of his figures gives a total for paraphrenia roughly similar to that found by Fenton, McGlashan and Heinssen (1988).

A possible additional source of paraphrenia cases is the increasing number of patients rather loosely diagnosed nowadays as 'schizoaffective'. Certainly, some of this author's clinical colleagues appear to be using that diagnosis not infrequently to describe a schizophrenia-like illness with well retained affect for which there is no satisfactory official category at present.

Risk factors

Predisposing factors which are generally mentioned include abnormal premorbid personality features, especially those characteristic of DSMIV cluster A personality disorders (Kendler, 1982), and peripheral sensory defects, especially deafness (Eastwood, Corbin and Reed, 1981) and, although to a lesser extent, visual loss (Guensberger, Fleischer and Sipkovska, 1977). Several researchers have agreed that patients with delusional-type disorders do not have a significant family history of schizophrenia, suggesting relative lack of a genetic link to schizophrenia (Munro, 1982; Watt, 1985).

Stability of the diagnosis

As already mentioned, Mayer (1921) found that approximately half of Kraepelin's patients with a diagnosis of paraphrenia eventually deteriorated to schizophrenia. Black, Yates and Andreasen (1988), on the other hand, state that 80 to 90 per cent of patients with delusional disorders (probably a mixture of paraphrenia and paranoia) remain diagnostically stable, and that their demographic characteristics differ markedly from patients with schizophrenia or a major mood disorder. As ever, it is difficult to know where the apparent statistics derive from, because of the lack of published research in the last three-quarters of a century, but one's impression is that indeed only a relatively small proportion of carefully diagnosed paraphrenic patients deteriorate to another disorder.

It should be emphasized that, until 40 years ago, *all* chronic schizophrenia-like psychoses tended to follow a deteriorative course, because of the lack of available treatments and the effects of long-term institutionalisation, so the end-state was not dissimilar whatever the original diagnosis. Nowadays, with treatment that is at least partly effective, that degree of degeneration is much less frequent, and good-outcome end-states are distinguishable from those with bad outcome. Clinical experience suggests, but cannot yet confirm, that individuals with paraphrenia are considerably more likely to be in the good prognosis group as compared with core schizophrenics.

Treatment

Paraphrenia appears to respond to most of the standard neuroleptic drugs, and no one medication is known to be more specifically efficacious than others. But it must again be stressed that there are no scientific data on this. Behavioural therapy may reduce the degree of preoccupation with the delusions shown by the patient (Kingdon, Tarkington and John, 1994). Psychotherapy may be a useful part of the rehabilitative process in re-covering treated patients but has not been shown to be of any value as a first-line treatment.

Treatment outcome

When the patient is collaborative with medication, the clinical outcome is frequently satisfactory. The patient becomes less anxious and agitated, is considerably less preoccupied with delusional thinking and with hallucinations, and is less likely to exhibit disturbed behaviour. As the illness improves, it is noticeable that affective warmth, appropriate mood responses and good rapport in interpersonal situations become increasingly prominent. This, in particular, distinguishes the paraphrenic patient from the paranoid schizophrenic, whose underlying personality is commonly stiff and humourless.

Unfortunately, in the noncompliant patient this degree of improvement is only glimpsed before relapse occurs and prognosis is likely to be as bad as in schizophrenia if lack of co-operation continues. In the older patient, even though the clinical outcome is reasonably good with consistent treatment, social outcome may be less satisfactory. Although the paraphrenic is relatively more sociable than other schizophrenics, the effects of a chronic psychiatric illness, increasing age-related problems, and relative difficulties with interpersonal relationships, may make rehabilitation in the community less satisfactory and the possibility of prolonged institutional care more likely.

Conclusion

If you do not expect the unexpected you will not find it.
Heraclitus (circa 500 BC)

A physician who has read this chapter and accepts the criteria proposed for paraphrenia will be able to recognize cases of this illness in his or her clinical practice. That, of itself, does not establish the validity of paraphrenia as a separate diagnosis, but it would certainly suggest that an informed approach allows one to differentiate its features from those of schizophrenia or delusional disorder. The question, then, is whether that differentiation has any practical value in terms of treatment and prognosis.

At this time it appears that the treatment of paranoid schizophrenia and paraphrenia are essentially similar but that the outcome in the latter may overall be better. However, to qualify that, there is a definite impression that paraphrenics are especially likely to be noncompliant with treatment in the long term, perhaps because their delusions remain persistent (Ravindran and Yatham, personal communication, 1997). Their relative emotional warmth and good rapport can disguise the ongoing existence of delusions, and may also mislead the therapist into thinking that co-operation with treatment is better than it is. Thus, when relapse occurs it may be unexpected and apparently sudden.

An accumulation of experience about paraphrenia conceptualised in modern terms is needed before we can begin to generalise about it. If it does prove to have worthwhile nosological qualities, it is predicted that it might become a more rational diagnostic niche for many schizophrenia-like cases which we cannot comfortably assign at this time. Should that be the case, not only would we have a more effective approach to these particular cases, but also we would have moved another step closer to making schizophrenia a less heterogeneous category.

Paranoid schizophrenia

Whatever one may say about its relationship to other schizophrenias or to delusional disorder, the actual diagnostic features of paranoid schizo-phrenia are relatively noncontroversial and can be studied in any standard textbook. The following brief account is provided mostly for complete-ness' sake but also as a counterpoint to the above description of para-phrenia.

As has been mentioned (p.156), Kraepelin included paranoid dementia praecox (subsequently paranoid schizophrenia) in his group of paranoid conditions along with paranoia (now delusional disorder) and paraph-renia. Nowadays, it is conventional to include it with other subtypes of schizophrenia but it has a number of features which distinguish it from them and this writer has, for many years, portrayed it as a bridge between delusional disorders and schizophrenia and as part of a paranoid spectrum (see p.156). For example, a family history of schizophrenia occurs only about half as often in paranoid schizophrenia as in other forms of schizo-phrenia, suggesting a much weaker genetic component (Farmer, McGuffin and Gottesman, 1985), and a number of authors, including Houlihan (1977) and Zigler and Glick (1984), have advanced strong arguments for considering it a separate disorder. Fuller Torrey (1981) has summarized the quite substantial epidemiological differences between paranoid and other schizophrenias.

Paranoid schizophrenia certainly shares many of the descriptive features of schizophrenia in general, but is particularly characterized by systematiz-ed, though not encapsulated, delusions and frequently by auditory halluci-nations. Probably persecutory delusions are most common, but somatic, jealousy and erotic themes are not infrequent, and all are commonly shot through with an element of disdain which frequently shades into grandio-sity. The hallucinations are often related to the predominant delusional themes. Tenseness, anxiety, agitation and anger often accompany the schizophrenic symptoms and there is a tendency for the patient to act out his anger and agitation with violence. Suicidal behaviour is not unknown. Severely disorganised behaviour and very flat or inappropriate affect are not unusual, but whereas paraphrenic individuals – even when psychotic – retain a good deal of emotional warmth and appropriate rapport, the paranoid schizophrenic tends to be stiff and distant in manner, and awkward and over-intense in relationship situations. Often, there is a coolness and unfeelingness mixed with the over-intensity.

Although the illness invades the personality and causes some degree of thought disorder, there is little incoherence. Some individuals may remain unrecognized and untreated in the community, although usually being thought of as eccentric and difficult, but such high functioning is relatively less common than in delusional disorders. Cognitive functions show little or no impairment. The following is a fairly typical example.

Case No. 13   Paranoid schizophrenia

The patient is a 48-year-old single, unemployed woman who has been admitted to a psychiatric hospital 30 times over a period of 22 years, on each occasion in almost identical circumstances. She has been diagnosed as schizophrenic since the age of 26 and for the past 15 years specifically as a paranoid schizophrenic.

She lives with elderly and ailing parents, but a brother who lives nearby accepts much of the responsibility for her supervision. The family are adamant that the patient should remain at home with them, although numerous attempts have been made to persuade them that she requires properly supervised community living. Admissions to hospital are invariably precipitated by the patient's stopping her medication: family members are usually aware of this but do nothing until her behaviour becomes disturbed and threatening. They then either bundle the patient into hospital or call the police to do this for them.

On admission, she is usually sullen and irritable and initially refuses to co-operate with treatment. She is suspicious of everybody and when she can get to a telephone she calls numerous people, including police, the ombudsman, a variety of physicians, local politicians and local government officials. To them she gives two very contradictory messages: first, that she is being unjustly held in hospital, and secondly that she wants an official order to be made requiring the police to kill her. She waylays medical and nursing staff incessantly in the hospital corridors, demanding to be allowed home, changes to medication and, frequently, a change of psychiatrist. At no time does she appear clinically depressed.

At interview when she is acutely unwell, her manner is angry and somewhat threatening. Speech is pressured, but conversation is stereotyped and repetitive. When not talking about her particular fixations, thinking is somewhat vague and irrelevant, and she expresses a variety of delusional ideas, many with a grandiose tinge. She admits to auditory hallucinations, usually voices talking about her unpleasantly in the third person or telling her to do certain things. She has no insight and insists she has no mental illness.

Sooner or later she always begins to accept neuroleptic treatment. She is currently on risperidone but has had many other antipsychotic drugs in the past. All of them seem to have approximately similar beneficial effects, in that over a period of 4–6 weeks her behaviour becomes better controlled, she is less irritable and she says the voices are less prominent, although they never entirely disappear. She stops telephoning and no longer asks that the police be authorised to kill her.

At her best she remains largely insightless. Her manner is stiff and humourless, and she has a secretive air, often with somewhat inappropriate sidelong glances and smiles. Nevertheless she is able to keep in touch with everyday affairs, look after her rather limited financial circumstances, and very effectively persuade her family to take her home yet again. Apart from one period of almost two years when she remained in relative remission, her admissions to hospital average about two per year. She has consistently refused to cooperate with any of the varied social supports which the mental health services have tried to provide for her and her family.

Paranoid schizophrenia tends to come on later than other schizophrenias and, in schizophrenias occurring for the first time in middle or old age, the appearances are most often those of the paranoid type. The later onset is usually cited as the reason for the better personality preservation since underlying personality features have had more time to develop and consolidate.

Treatment is, as in other forms of schizophrenia and paraphrenia, with neuroleptics. The clinical response to treatment is often good: for example, Pearlson and colleagues, (1989) reported that almost a half of their elderly schizophrenics – most with the paranoid type – did excellently on treatment. Unfortunately, in practice, many fail to retain their improvement because of poor social supports and poor treatment compliance. Quite often, the patient retains marked ideas of reference: this, plus an inappropriate degree of self-confidence, persuades him or her that psychiatric treatment is not required and so the medication is sooner or later discarded. A proportion of patients with paranoid schizophrenia therefore has a pattern of repeated breakdowns and readmissions.

Paranoid schizophrenia should be delineated from other schizophrenias and should never be confused with paranoia/delusional disorder. In clinical work, the distinction from paraphrenia may be less important as treatment and prognosis are similar, but in research on paranoid schizophrenia, cases of paraphrenia should be clearly separated since their aetiology and prognosis, as has been mentioned, may be significantly different.

References

Anderson, E.W. and Trethowan, W.H. (1973). *Psychiatry*, 3rd edn. p. 165. London: Baillière Tindall.
Arieti, S. (1955). *Interpretation of Schizophrenia*, p. 11. New York: Brunner Mazel.
Black, D.W., Yates, W.R. and Andreasen, N.C. (1988). Delusional (paranoid) disorders. In *Textbook of Psychiatry*, ed. J.A. Talbott, pp. 391–396. Washington, DC: American Psychiatric Association.
Bleuler, E. (1950). *Dementia Praecox or The Group of Schizophrenias*, transl. J. Zinkin New York: International Universities Press.
Brink, T.L., Capri, D., Deneeve, V., Janakes, C. and Oliveira, C. (1979). Hypochondriasis and paranoia: similar delusional systems in an institutionalized geriatric population. *J. Nerv. Ment. Dis.* 167: 224–228.
Curran, D. and Partridge, M. (1969). *Psychological Medicine*, 6th edn, p. 190. Edinburgh: Livingstone.
Diagnostic and Statistical Manual of Mental Disorders, 3rd edn. (DSMIII) (1980). Washington, DC: American Psychiatric Association.
Diagnostic and Statistical Manual of Mental Disorders, 3rd edn. revised (DSMIIIR) (1987). Washington, DC: American Psychiatric Association.
Diagnostic and Statistical Manual of Mental Disorders, 4th edn. (DSMIV) (1994). Washington, DC: American Psychiatric Association.
Eastwood, R., Corbin, S. and Reed, M. (1981). Hearing impairment and paraphrenia. *J. Otolaryngol.* 10: 306–308.
Farmer, A.E., McGuffin, P. and Gottesman, I.I. (1985). Searching for the split in schizophrenia: a twin study perspective. *Psychiat. Res.* 13: 109–118.
Fenton, W.S., McGlashan, T.H. and Heinssen, R.K. (1988). A comparison of DSMIII and DSMIIIR schizophrenia. *Am. J. Psychiat.* 145: 1446–1449.
Fish, F.J. (1964). *An Outline of Psychiatry*, p. 116. Bristol: John Wright and Sons.

Fuller Torrey, E. (1981). The epidemiology of paranoid schizophrenia. *Schizophr. Bull.* **7**: 588–593.

Guensberger, E., Fleischer, J. and Sipkovska, E. (1977). On the psychopathology of paranoid psychosis in the blind. *Cesk. Psychiatr.* **73**: 291–296.

Gurland, B.J., Fleiss, J.L., Cooper, J.E., Sharpe, L., Kendell, R.E. and Roberts, P. (1970). Cross-national study of diagnosis of mental disorders: hospital diagnoses and hospital patients in New York and London. *Compr. Psychiat.* **11**: 18–25.

Harris, M.J. and Jeste, D.V. (1988). Late-onset schizophrenia: an overview. *Schizophr. Bull.* **14**: 39–55.

Henderson, D. and Batchelor, I.R. (1962). *Henderson and Gillespie's Textbook of Psychiatry*, 9th edn. London: Oxford University Press.

Houlihan, J.P. (1977). Heterogeneity among schizophrenic patients: selective review of recent findings (1970–75). *Schizophr. Bull.* **3**: 246–258.

International Statistical Classification of Diseases, 9th revision (ICD9) (1978). Geneva: World Health Organization.

International Statistical Classification of Diseases, 10th revision (ICD10) (1992–93) Geneva: World Health Organization.

Jette, C.C.B. and Winnett, R.L. (1987). Late-onset paranoid disorder. *Am. J. Orthopsychiat.* **57**: 485–494.

Kendler, K.S. (1982). Demography of paranoid psychosis (delusional disorder). *Arch. Gen. Psychiat.* **39**: 890–902.

Kingdon, D., Tarkington, D. and John, C. (1994). Cognitive behaviour therapy of schizophrenia. *Br. J. Psychiat.* **164**: 581–587.

Kolb, L.C. (1973). *Modern Clinical Psychiatry*, 8th edn, p. 389. Philadelphia: W. B. Saunders.

Kolle, K. (1931). *Die Primäre Verücktheit: Psychopathologische, Klinische und Genealogische Untersuchungen*. Leipzig:Thieme.

Kraepelin, E. (1909–13). *Lehrbuch der Psychiatrie*, 8th edn. Leipzig: Barth.

Kraepelin, E. (1921). *Manic-Depressive Insanity and Paranoia*. transl. R.M. Barclay, (1976). New York: Arno Press.

Leigh, D., Pare, C.M.B. and Marks, J. (1977). *A Concise Encyclopaedia of Psychiatry*, p. 273. Lancaster, England: MTP Press.

Leonhard, K. (1960). Die Atypischen Psychosen und Kleists Lehre von den Endogenen Psychosen In *Psychiatrie der Gegenwart*, ed. H. Gruhle, Vol. 2. Berlin: Springer.

Lewis, A. (1970). Paranoia and paranoid: a historical perspective. *Psychol. Med.* **1**: 2–12.

Mayer, W. (1921). Über paraphrene Psychosen. *Z. Ges. Neurol. Psychiat.* **71**: 187–206.

Merskey, H. (1980). *Psychiatric Illness*, 3rd edn., p. 102. London: Baillière Tindall.

Munro, A. (1982). *Delusional Hypochondriasis*. Clarke Institute of Psychiatry Monograph No. 5. Toronto: Clarke Institute of Psychiatry.

Munro, A. (1989). Classification of patients not meeting DSMIIIR criteria for schizophrenia. *Am. J. Psychiat.* **146**: 816–817(letter).

Munro, A. (1991). A plea for paraphrenia. *Can. J. Psychiat.* **36**: 667–672.

Pearlson, G.D., Kreger, L., Rabins, P.V., Chase, G.A., Cohen, B., Wirth, J.B., Schlaepfer, T.B. and Tune, L.E. (1989). A chart review study of late-onset and early-onset schizophrenia. *Am. J. Psychiat.* **146**: 1568–1574.

Roth, M. (1955). The natural history of mental disorder in old age. *J. Ment. Sci.* **101**: 281–301.

Sullivan, H.S. (1962). *Schizophrenia as a Human Process*, p. 16. New York: W.W. Norton.

Watt, J.A.G. (1985). The relationship of paranoid states to schizophrenia. *Am. J. Psychiat.* **145**: 1456–1458.

Williams, J.B.W. (1987). Psychotic and mood disorders. *Hosp. Commun. Psychiat.* **38**: 13–14.

Zigler, E. and Glick, M. (1984). Paranoid schizophrenia: an unorthodox view. *Am. J. Orthopsychiat* **54**: 43–70.

8
'Late' paraphrenia and late onset schizophrenia

Introduction

Schizophrenia often occurs at an early age and the patient can then live well into old age, displaying persistent psychotic symptoms of various sorts. This is not controversial. However, the idea that schizophrenia could appear for the first time in middle age or among the elderly has been the subject of considerable argument for many years.

Nowadays there seems to be much wider acceptance that schizophrenia-like illnesses can originate at any time from the teens onwards. It appears that, the older the age of onset, the more will the case resemble paranoid schizophrenia and the less significant will be the genetic component. Unhappily, there are still arguments, often based on ideological rather than scientific grounds, as to whether late onset cases should be regarded as schizophrenia or as something else (Stoudemire and Riether, 1987).

In the recent past, it has become common in the United States to diagnose schizophrenia of first onset in the elderly. This also happens to some extent in the United Kingdom, but notable arguments continue there about the differentiation of late paraphrenia from old-age schizophrenia. It probably makes little difference to the type of treatment which is applied if the case is called one or the other. However, if late paraphrenia is indeed paraphrenia as described in Chapter 7, but simply coming on for the first time in older age, then its prognosis might be somewhat better than that of a case of schizophrenia, at least in the short- to mid-term (Naguib, 1991). The problem is that, the older the patient, the more difficult it is to make a clinical distinction between a 'late' paraphrenia and a 'late' schizophrenia on clinical grounds, and perhaps such a distinction is relatively unimportant at that stage.

In the case which will shortly be described, the individual could be regarded as having exhibited schizoid tendencies for much of his life, yet he had a successful career and a stable marriage and he only became psychiatrically ill after his wife's death. Some psychiatrists would undoubtedly regard him as suffering from late-onset schizophrenia, but as the features of 'late' paraphrenia are unfolded subsequently in this chapter, the reader will perhaps see why a diagnosis of paraphrenia is preferred here. In this writer's view, there is no need to describe the case as one of 'late' paraphrenia, since the situation is simply one in which a relatively typical paraphrenia develops in an older person.

Case No. 14 Paraphrenia originating in older age

A childless man aged 74 had had a successful career, although he had always been regarded as aloof and had few social activities outside the home. He retired at the age of 62 and for several years appeared happy, mostly in the company of his wife. When he was 67, his wife died of cancer and he took this very badly: in fact, his family physician treated him for a time with an antidepressant. Thereafter, he increasingly secluded himself. He would be seen tending his small garden or making brief trips to the local shops, but he would conspicuously avoid talking to neighbours or others. Local people began to be offended because he would shout at children who strayed into his garden, frightening the smaller ones, and he would confiscate balls and toys which came over the garden wall.

Unfortunately, his house caught fire one night and was badly damaged: apparently the fire was purely accidental. He was found wandering in the garden in a dazed state and was taken to hospital. There, he was noted to have slight effects of smoke inhalation but was otherwise physically intact. However, he was thought to be 'confused' and was subsequently admitted as a psychiatric inpatient. On the psychiatric unit he was found to be very agitated and he made various wild statements about his neighbours persecuting him and burning his house down. He was not clinically confused and neurological investigations were consistently normal. He was treated with adequate doses of neuroleptic medication and the distress settled, but the persecutory beliefs remained. They were wide-ranging, and involved police and local government as well as neighbours. A nephew, giving a collateral history, stated that he had heard his uncle expressing these beliefs for several years, often with much associated anger, and the nephew was adamant that the beliefs were unfounded.

The patient gradually settled and was transferred to a psychogeriatric unit where there was an active rehabilitation programme. He was again found to be cognitively and intellectually intact, but his multiple delusions, though muted, remained. Although a very reserved and 'private' individual, he was pleasant and emotionally appropriate while on medication. Subsequently, with some reluctance, the nephew and his wife agreed to have the patient in their home for a trial period, but within days he stopped taking his neuroleptic and relapsed into being angry, unpleasant and accusatory. He is now in a residential home for the elderly where his medication is supervised. He remains pleasant and marginally sociable, but still extremely deluded. Staff report that at times he behaves as though he may be listening to auditory hallucinations.

Let us now briefly consider some of the issues relating to the diagnosis of 'late' paraphrenia and schizophrenia of late onset.

'Late' paraphrenia

This diagnostic category originated in the United Kingdom and is used quite widely there, in Europe and in parts of the British Commonwealth, but it has never received official recognition in North America. As Almeida and colleagues (1992a) note, even in parts of the world where it was utilized it appears to be losing its currency, and late paraphrenia is not included in either ICD10 or DSMIV, although these authors still find some use for the concept.

Roth and Morrissey (1952) introduced the term to describe a group of elderly individuals who had well organised delusions and hallucinations in the setting of well preserved personality features and good affective response. Later, Kay and Roth (1961) expanded this to include all elderly patients with a paranoid illness which was not primary affective disorder, delirium or dementia. Delusions were most commonly persecutory but could be hypochondriacal, erotic or grandiose.

As one reads these descriptions now, it is often difficult to know whether individual cases would be diagnosed in latter-day terms as delusional disorder, paraphrenia (as defined in Chapter 7) or schizophrenia of late onset, and early on there were criticisms that late paraphrenia was more likely a heterogeneous group of nonaffective, nondemented delusional illnesses arising in the over-60 age group (Fish, 1960; Holden, 1987). Also early on, there was a perception that there might be significant organic brain dysfunction involved even if these patients were not demented (Herbert and Jacobson, 1967), a situation very similar to that in late onset schizophrenia.

In the 1950s and 1960s, it was conventionally believed that schizophrenia rarely had its onset after the age of 45, and it was therefore all but impossible to diagnose schizophrenia of late onset. Late paraphrenia allowed the psychiatrist to diagnose a schizophrenia-like functional psychosis of late life without actually calling it schizophrenia and was very useful in separating out a group of older patients with certain common features. But the suspicion of heterogeneity has not been allayed (Quintal, Day-Cody and Levy, 1991). Kay and Roth (1961) and Post (1966) attempted to define subgroups which, in fact, did not seem to retain cohesiveness over time; Holden (1987) modified this approach and, after excluding organic and mood disorders, found cases corresponding to schizophreniform, schizoaffective and delusional disorders, suggesting again a mixture of diagnostic types.

Most elderly people do not develop paranoid symptoms or hallucinations (Corbin and Eastwood, 1986) and there have been many attempts to find reasons why a minority should become paranoid in old age. Traditionally there have been reports of an excess of over-sensitive, paranoid or schizoid premorbid personality traits, but some of the difficulties in assessing these retrospectively have been noted elsewhere (see pp.58–59). Deafness and other sensory deficits as isolating factors are often cited, but again may be difficult to quantify, although Eastwood, Corbin and Reed (1981) and Khan, Clark and Oyebode (1988) appear to show that application of a hearing aid may considerably reduce paranoid beliefs and behaviour in hearing-compromised individuals with psychotic symptoms. Social isolation for whatever reason is widely regarded as a provoking factor in delusional illness of the elderly but as Almeida and colleagues (1992b) point out, it can also prevent recognition of the illness in a proportion of cases because no one gets near enough to the patient to appreciate its presence.

Modern technologies, such as CT scanning, magnetic resonance imaging (MRI) and others have begun to shed considerable new light on delusional/paranoid illnesses in the elderly. Miller and colleagues (1986 and 1991) compared a group of patients suffering from later onset psychosis with healthy controls: they found that the former had an excess of white-matter lesions or metabolic illnesses, and performed more poorly on tests of frontal lobe and memory function. Breitner and colleagues (1990) and Förstl and colleagues (1991) have also reported white-matter lesions, and the latter comment that it is possible that a combination of subcortical abnormality with an intact cortex may be a neuropathological basis for certain types of delusions.

Flint, Rifat and Eastwood (1991) divided cases into late paraphrenia and late onset paranoia (i.e. delusional disorder) groups and reported a much higher frequency of hitherto unsuspected cerebral infarction in the paranoia patients as shown by CT scanning. Howard and colleagues (1992) examined the brains of 41 individuals with late paraphrenia and found that those who had had Schneiderian first-rank symptoms showed significantly less atrophy of the cerebral cortex. Levy (1990) noted that he and his colleagues found that there was a marked contrast between early onset schizophrenia, in which few patients demonstrated enlarged lateral ventricles, and late onset schizophrenia, where enlarged ventricles were common. Howard and colleagues (1992) stress that the lesions in late paraphrenia are different from those in Alzheimer's dementia and, though the patients may show some cognitive and memory deficits, these are not at the level of dementia.

The situation is still in a state of flux and attempts to correlate clinical subtypes with specific neuropathological findings remain at a tentative level as yet (Addonizio, 1995). Nevertheless, we seem to be seeing the beginning of a trend, the first element of which is the increasing certainty that late paraphrenia is indeed a heterogeneous group. Miller and colleagues (1991) use the general term 'late life psychosis' which is virtually equivalent to late paraphrenia, and suggest that late onset schizophrenia is one subgroup of this.

Another element in the trend is the increasing attempt to distinguish schizophrenia, paraphrenia and paranoia/delusional disorder in the elderly, and the finding by Flint, Rifat and Eastwood (1991) of more cerebral pathology in delusional disorder as compared with paraphrenia, is both interesting and surprising, as is the linking of Schneiderian first-rank symptoms to nonatrophy of the brain (Howard and colleagues, 1992). Yassa and Suranyi-Cadotte (1993) have clinically separated subgroups of late onset schizophrenia (20 subjects), paraphrenia (7 subjects) and delusional disorder without hallucinations (13 subjects), and have itemised their main clinical characteristics. They find that the schizophrenics have bizarre delusions, auditory hallucinations and some tendency to Schneiderian first-rank symptoms and negative symptomatology; paraphrenics (who, in this study, may in fact be hallucinated delusional disorder patients) have predominantly nonbizarre delusions, auditory hallucinations, an earlier onset, and premorbid paranoid or schizoid personality disorder: delusional disorder without hallucinations has a later onset, nonbizarre delusions, a relatively normal premorbid personality and (often) an underlying physical illness.

Bridge and Wyatt (1980a and b) stated that late paraphrenia was often misdiagnosed or overlooked in the United States. It seems increasingly clear that diagnostic confusion within the category is relatively common and it is losing its popularity as a result. Schizophrenia of late onset is now a respectable diagnosis in DSMIV and ICD10: as Almeida and colleagues (1992a) comment, we do not yet know whether the same underlying aetiological factors apply to early as to late schizophrenia but, as we have seen, there is growing consensus that as the age of onset increases, genetic factors decrease in importance and organic brain factors become more significant.

Conclusion

The present author's thesis is that there is an age continuum not only for schizophrenia but for delusional disorder and also paraphrenia. These two delusional disorders can arise, it seems, at any adult age and it appears likely that, as with schizophrenia, brain pathology plays a greater and greater role the older the age of onset. As noted, there are indications that authors are – albeit still imperfectly – moving towards accepting these categories in elderly patients, and we may be seeing the very beginning of correlations between the clinical pictures and the underlying neuropathological changes. It is again suggested that the term 'late paraphrenia' is now redundant and, if used at all, should simply denote a case of paraphrenia which appears to have arisen for the first time in an older person.

At the clinical level, it appears that, the older the patient, the closer are the similarities between late onset paraphrenia and late onset schizophrenia, with regard to neuropathology and to treatment and prognosis. In the very old, there may be little value in trying to make the differentiation and this writer's preference would be to opt for a diagnosis of late onset schizophrenia in these circumstances.

On the other hand, we are probably on the threshold of differentiating a number of clinical subgroups amongst elderly patients with first onset schizophrenia-like illnesses, but advances in this area are increasingly being made with the aid of technological interventions, not as a result of clinical speculation.

Schizophrenia of late onset

As has been noted elsewhere, Kraepelin accepted that schizophrenia could appear for the first time in middle or old age but perhaps his term 'dementia praecox' (precocious dementia) overemphasized the undoubted tendency for most cases of schizophrenia to appear in earlier life. Whatever the reason, by the mid-twentieth century Fish (1960) wrote that it was unusual in the Anglo-American psychiatric literature to find a psychiatric illness designated as schizophrenia if it had begun after the age of 40, and he noted that it was usual to call chronic paranoid psychoses occurring in middle or later life 'paranoid states' or 'paraphrenia'. As recorded in the preceding section on late paraphrenia, such terms were partly to avoid an ideological argument and to allow workers to recognize later-life schizophrenia-like illness without being ridiculed for calling it schizophrenia. However, a gradually increasing pressure developed to call a spade a spade and, by 1972, Kay (a proponent of late paraphrenia) stated that chronic paranoid hallucinatory states which arise late in life were schizophrenia from a descriptive point of view. He thought there was a continuum from schizophrenia of earlier onset but again emphasized that, the older the patient, the more likely was it that organic cerebral pathology would play a significant part.

By the 1980s, there was a definite trend, especially in the American literature, to accept the concept of late onset schizophrenia (Rabins, Pauker and Thomas, 1984; Jeste and colleagues, 1988), and Harris and Jeste (1988) provided an authoritative overview of the evidence to that date. Templer (1989) emphasized the largely semantic difficulties in making the diagnosis of schizophrenia of late onset, and there was a growing campaign to persuade DSM and ICD to accept the concept. Pearlson and colleagues (1989) compared late onset with early onset cases and found many similarities, but also noted that the older individuals had more visual, tactile and olfactory hallucinations and a larger number of different types of hallucination, with a greater tendency to persecutory delusions and premorbid schizoid personality traits. On the other hand, younger patients showed more thought disorder and more affective flattening. Visual and auditory impairment due to physical causes, not surprisingly, were more common in the elderly. In terms of treatment, almost half of the older patients responded excellently to treatment with neuroleptics. Rabins and colleagues (1987) showed that the lateral cerebral ventricles in late onset schizophrenia were larger than in early onset cases but significantly smaller than in Alzheimer's disease, a finding which has been repeatedly confirmed since.

An interesting additional factor relates to gender and the age of onset of schizophrenia. Seeman and Lang (1990) reported that female schizophrenics were likely to experience a later onset on average than males, but that after the menopause they showed an excess rate of onset of schizophrenia; speculation on the possible quasi-neuroleptic effects of oestrogens is still ongoing. Flor-Henry (1990) found that the later the onset of schizophrenia the greater was the excess of females, even allowing for differential death rates between men and women at that age, and this remains a robust finding.

DSMIV and ICD10 have now eliminated an upper age limit for the onset of schizophrenia and there is increasing acquiescence with the idea of diagnosing first onset schizophrenia right into extreme old age. However, some psychiatrists are still uncertain about this and continue to diagnose such cases as late paraphrenia or even, at times, delusional disorder. As suggested on p.173, the separate diagnosis of late paraphrenia is probably not justifiable nowadays and we have seen that delusional disorder has its own set of quite separate criteria. If an elderly patient develops a schizophrenia-like illness for the first time, the diagnosis should be schizophrenia, other things being equal. The presence of organic brain factors is no deterrent to the diagnosis unless the organic disease is of such degree as to warrant an entirely separate recognition.

Conclusion

To be as simplistic as possible, one might say that paraphrenia and schizophrenia can each originate at any age from the teens onward, and a first onset of either disorder is perfectly possible in the elderly. On the other hand, attempts to sustain a separate diagnostic category of late paraphrenia have proven increasingly unconvincing and the category seems to be at best a mixed one. In the most elderly, a clinical differentiation of late onset paraphrenia from late onset schizophrenia, especially of the paranoid type, may be impracticable and, in any case, new forms of investigation are demonstrating various neuropathological abnormalities in such patients which may become the basis in the future for an entirely different classification of 'paranoid' illnesses in the senium.

If one could confidently make a diagnosis of paraphrenia in an elderly patient, utilising the criteria set out in Chapter 9, then the patient's illness is paraphrenia, not 'late' paraphrenia.

References

Addonizio, G.C. (1995). Late paraphenia. *Psychiat. Clin. N. Am.* **18**: 335–344.

Almeida, O.P., Howard, R., Förstl, H. and Levy, R. (1992a). Should the diagnosis of late paraphrenia be abandoned? *Psychol. Med.* **22**: 11–14.

Almeida, O.P., Howard, R., Förstl, H. and Levy, R. (1992b) Late paraphrenia: a review. *Int. J. Geriat. Psychiat.* **7**: 543–548.

Breitner, J.C.S., Husain, M.M. Figiel, G.S., Krishnan, K.R.R. and Boyko, O.B. (1990). Cerebral white matter disease in late-onset paranoid psychosis. *Biol. Psychiat.* **28**: 266–274.

Bridge, T.P. and Wyatt, R.J. (1980a). Paraphrenia: paranoid states of late life. I. European research. *J. Am. Geriat. Soc.* **28**: 193–200.

Bridge, T.P. and Wyatt, R.J. (1980b). Paraphrenia: paranoid states of late life. II. American research. *J. Am. Geriat. Soc.* **28**: 201–205.

Corbin, S.L. and Eastwood, M.R. (1986). Sensory deficits and mental disorders of old age: causal or coincidental associations? *Psychol. Med.* **16**: 251–256.

Eastwood, M.R., Corbin, S. and Reed, M. (1981). Hearing impairment and paraphrenia. *J. Otolaryng.* **10**: 306–308.

Fish, F. (1960). Senile schizophrenia. *J. Ment. Sci.* **106**: 938–946.

Flint, A.J., Rifat, S.L. and Eastwood, M.R. (1991). Late-onset paranoia: distinct from paraphrenia? *Int. J. Geriat. Psychiat.* **6**: 103–109.

Flor-Henry, P. (1990). Influence of gender in schizophrenia as related to other psychopathological syndromes. *Schizophren. Bull.* **16**: 211–227.

Förstl, H., Howard, R., Almeida, O., Burns, A., Naguib, M. and Levy, R. (1991). Cranial computed tomography findings – late paraphrenia with and without FRS. *Nervenarzt* **62**: 274–276.

Harris, M.J. and Jeste, D.V. (1988). Late-onset schizophrenia: an overview. *Schizophren. Bull.* **14**: 39–55.

Herbert, M.E. and Jacobson, S. (1967). Late paraphrenia. *Br. J. Psychiat.* **113**: 461–469.

Holden, N.L. (1987). Late paraphrenia or the paraphrenias? A descriptive study with a 10–year follow-up. *Br. J. Psychiat.* **150**: 635–639.

Howard, R.J., Förstl, H., Naguib, M., Burns, A. and Levy, R. (1992). First-rank symptoms of Schneider in late paraphrenia. Cortical structural correlates. *Br. J. Psychiat.* **160**: 108–109.

Jeste, D.J., Harris, M.J., Pearlson, G.D., Rabins, P., Lesser, I., Miller, B., Coles, C. and Yassa, R. (1988). Late-onset schizophrenia. Studying clinical validity. *Psychiat. Clin. N. Am.* **11**: 1–13.

Kay, D.W.K. (1972). Schizophrenia and schizophrenia-like states in the elderly. *Br. J. Hosp. Med.* **8**: 369–376.

Kay, D.W.K. and Roth, M. (1961). Environmental and hereditary factors in the schizophrenias of old age ('late paraphrenia') and their bearing on the general problem of causation in schizophrenia. *J. Ment. Sci.* **107**: 649–686.

Khan, A.M., Clark, T. and Oyebode, F. (1988). Unilateral auditory hallucinations. *Br. J. Psychiat.* **152**: 297–298 (letter).

Levy, R. (1990). Late-onset and early-onset schizophrenia. *Am. J. Psychiat.* **147**: 1382–1383 (letter).

Miller, B.L., Benson, D.F., Cummings, J.L. and Neshkes, R. (1986). Late-life paraphrenia: an organic delusional syndrome. *J. Clin. Psychiat.* **47**: 204–207.

Miller, B.L., Lesser, I.M., Boone, K.B., Hill, E., Mehringer, C.M. and Wong, K. (1991). Brain lesions and cognitive function in late life psychosis. *Br. J. Psychiat.* **158**: 76–82.

Naguib, M. (1991). Paraphrenia revisited. *Br. J. Hosp. Med.* **46**: 371–375.

Pearlson, G.D., Kreger, L., Rabins, P.V., Chase, G.A., Cohen, B., Wirth, J.B., Schlaepfer, T.B. and Tune, L.E. (1989). A chart review study of late-onset and early-onset schizophrenia. *Am. J. Psychiat.* **146**: 1568–1574.

Post, F. (1966). *Persistent Persecutory States of the Elderly.* Oxford: Pergamon Press.

Quintal, M., Day-Cody, D. and Levy, R. (1991). Late paraphrenia and ICD10. *Int. J. Geriat. Psychiat.* **6**: 111–116.

Rabins, P., Pauker, S. and Thomas, J. (1984). Can schizophrenia begin after age 44? *Comp. Psychiat.* **25**: 290–294.

Rabins, P., Pearlson, G., Jayaram, G., Steele, C. and Tune, L. (1987). Increased ventricle-to-brain ratio in late-onset schizophrenia. *Am. J. Psychiat* **144**: 1216–1218.

Roth, M. and Morrissey, J. (1952). Problems in the diagnosis and classification of mental disorders in old age. *J. Ment. Sci.* **98**: 66–80.

Seeman, M.V. and Lang, M. (1990). The role of estrogens in schizophrenia gender differences. *Schizophren. Bull.* **16**: 185–194.

Stoudemire, A. and Riether, A.M. (1987). Evaluation and treatment of paranoid syndromes in the elderly: a review. *Gen. Hosp. Psychiat.* **9**: 267–274.

Templer, D.I. (1989). A comment on late-onset schizophrenia. *Schizophren. Bull.* **15**: 173–174 (letter).

Yassa, R. and Suranyi-Cadotte, B. (1993). Clinical characteristics of late-onset schizophrenia and delusional disorder. *Schizophren. Bull.* **19**: 701–707.

9
Delusional misidentification syndrome (DMS)

This group of disorders is characterized by delusions of misidentification, often accompanied by hallucinations of misidentification (Debruille and Stip, 1996). There are relatively 'pure' forms in which the delusion forms the greater part of the presentation and similar pictures in which the delusion is secondary to other disorders, such as schizophrenia, severe depression or Alzheimer's disease (Spier, 1992). In the past, cases have often been misdiagnosed as schizophrenia (Ellis and Young, 1990).

There are four main variants and experts in the field describe additional alternative forms of these. The types most commonly mentioned are:

(1) The Capgras syndrome (Capgras and Reboul-Lachaux, 1923), in which the patient perceives someone in his environment (usually a closely related individual) to have been replaced by an almost, but not quite, exact double.
(2) The Frégoli syndrome (Courbon and Fail, 1927) where the patient believes that persecutors have altered their facial appearance to resemble familiar people in the environment.
(3) Intermetamorphosis (Courbon and Tusques, 1932), in which the patient thinks that the people around him or her have changed identities with each other, so that A becomes B, B becomes C, and so on.
(4) Subjective doubles (Christodoulou, 1978) where the patient believes that exact doubles of him- or herself exist. This is said usually to co-exist with other forms of DMS and is rarely seen by itself.

The terminology in this area is almost as confusing as in the delusional disorders, and de Pauw (1994a) has made a strong plea for rationalisation of the nomenclature, while suggesting a classification according to the type of altered recognition experienced by the patient and by known aetiological factors.

Hypothesized psychodynamic factors in DMS

Relatively early in the career of DMS, when neuropathological formulations were still unavailable, attempts to explain the disorder's phenomena in psychological terms were dominated by psychoanalytic theories. These are best summarized by Berson (1983) who proposes that, since DMS usually involves significant others, there is already intense affect towards these. When the feelings become too ambivalent to tolerate, psychological splitting occurs and projection (as in paranoia) is employed. The original person becomes all good and the impostor all bad which safeguards the internal economy of the psyche but is not, in practice, an effective coping mechanism. As de Pauw (1994b) has pointed out, all of this is totally speculative and is seriously undercut by the increasing recognition of actual brain pathology in a high proportion of cases. Allied to this is the fact that the patients tend to be older than one would expect for an illness of mainly psychological aetiology. It has to be accepted at this time that psychodynamic formulations of DMS have extremely limited value in the assessment and treatment of the disorder.

The DMSs currently have no official niche in our psychiatric classifications, and elsewhere (Munro, 1995) the present author has proposed that they should properly belong to an expanded category of delusional disorders in DSMIV and ICD10. Spier (1992) implies that they belong there when he refers to them along with 'other types of paranoia', and Manschrek (1992), a distinguished figure in the field of delusional disorders, obviously agreed with this when he included Spier's article on DMSs in the May 1992 edition of *Psychiatric Annals* which is devoted entirely to delusional disorders.

As has been noted repeatedly in this book, delusions occur in many psychiatric disorders, but the term 'delusional disorder' is restricted to the illness described as such in DSMIV and ICD10. Similarly, as stated, DMS can apparently be a syndrome in its own right or can be a symptom occurring in the setting of other psychiatric disorders. This writer's general contention is that the free-standing syndrome is the one to be designated as an additional delusional disorder. The symptomatic cases belong with their parent disorders.

However, the situation is not altogether that simple. Now that an increasing proportion of cases has been shown to have organic brain correlates (Anderson, 1988; Doran, 1990), this gives rise to classificatory difficulties. For example, if an absolutely typical DMS occurs which seems to be totally unrelated to other major psychiatric disorders but has been shown to be associated with some demonstrable brain dysfunction, could it still be admitted to the category of delusional disorder?

In fact, a similar problem has already been addressed in relation to the delusional disorders (see p.61). In a proportion of cases of paranoia/delusional disorder there is a demonstrated or inferred organic brain factor (Munro, 1982), but if this is at a relatively subtle level and is not producing evidence of an actual organic mental disorder, then the case can be accepted as a delusional disorder. (And there is evidence that these cases respond similarly to psychotropic treatment, as compared with the 'functional' cases.)

It seems to the present author that a similar approach could be adopted with the DMSs. If the DMS is present, the presence or absence of an organic brain factor can be specified. If the organic factor is moderate, the case should be classified with the delusional disorders. If the organic factor is sufficiently severe that another disorder (for example, Alzheimer type dementia) is recognized, the case belongs with that other disorder's category.

Features of DMS

DMS occurs in both sexes and across a wide age range, but especially in the middle aged and elderly. Weinstein (1994) makes some interesting points about the disorder's features, for example:

(1) The misidentification is not indiscriminate. A limited number of people, places or objects is involved, and these are often closely familiar to the sufferer.

(2) There is an intriguing mixture of misidentification and, at the same time, implicit recognition of the identity of the person, place or object.

(3) There is frequently an admixture of depersonalisation and derealisation (often particularly noticeable at the onset of symptoms).

(4) The individual's own reaction to the misidentification situation will often be coloured by psychological factors from his or her background.

(5) Although the variants are described as separate entities, there is often overlap of features from more than one type in particular cases.

Spier (1992) points out that the disorder is not as rare as was previously believed and there is a steady trickle of new case-descriptions in the current psychiatric literature, although not every article makes clear whether it is describing the DMS syndrome or the DMS symptom secondary to another psychiatric illness. The same author notes some particularly important features of the syndrome:

(1) There is a considerable potential for violence. Many of these patients feel persecuted and believe that the substitution of identity is done to harm them. They may become enraged and attack the 'fraud', who is usually someone close to them, quite often in a dangerous fashion (Silva and colleagues, 1992).
(2) The presence of a DMS symptom complex makes the prognosis of any other co-existing psychiatric disorder worse.
(3) Since there is growing evidence for organic abnormalities in the brain as significant aetiological factors (Fishbain, 1987), the recognition of DMS should alert the physician to the possible presence of brain disease.

There are now many reports on brain abnormalities in DMS, based predominantly on single cases or on very short series. There seems to be a consensus that disorders of the right cerebral hemisphere are especially likely to occur: Spier (1992) mentions the right temporo-parietal area as particularly suspect but not yet proven, and other authors also emphasize right-sided lesions (de Pauw, Szulecka and Poltock, 1987; Ellis and Young, 1990; Förstl and colleagues, 1991; Fleminger and Burns, 1993). However, there are reports of damage to other brain areas in relation to DMS, and Joseph (1986) and Signer(1994) provide examples of this.

What is especially interesting is that, whatever the exact location of the brain dysfunction, at least two-thirds of cases of DMS have some demonstrable lesion which may well have a casual connection with the misidentification symptoms. This allows for speculation about factors operating in normal and abnormal face recognition, which are especially related to operation of the right cerebral hemisphere (Ellis, 1994), and to mechanisms for relating sensory information to the appropriate affective response, a process which is impaired in DMS (Ellis and Young, 1990; Weinstein, 1994). Brugger, Monsch and Johnson (1996) note that the right cerebral hemisphere appears to be dominant for suppression of repetitive behaviour and lesions there may result in inability to moderate behaviour (and presumably the associated belief systems), a feature typical of all delusional presentations.

McAllister (1992), basing his speculations on the work of Cummings (1985), Landis and colleagues (1986),Van Lancker and colleagues (1988), Gorman and Cummings (1990), and others, has suggested that malfunction of limbic–basal ganglia mechanisms is involved in the genesis of delusions, with special emphasis on dopamine overactivity. He recognizes what appears to be an important contribution of right parieto-occipital lobe abnormalities to the specific syndrome of misidentification and hypothesises a disintegration in the complex interaction of cortex, limbic system and basal ganglia in generating Capgras and related phenomena. Ten years earlier the present author (Munro, 1982) put forward the possibility of a locus of circumscribed abnormal brain function in paranoia/ delusional disorder, most likely in the temporal lobe/limbic area and also involving dopamine overactivity. Elsewhere, there is evidence linking limbic lobe abnormalities with 'paranoid symptoms' (Onuma, 1983). An elaboration of these observations could suggest a complex brain system, perhaps integrating sensory and affective data and involving a mechanism to down-regulate repetitive behaviour, whose malfunction results in delusions. The nature and particular content of the delusion would be determined by the specific site within the system at which the predominance of abnormal activity was taking place. This paradigm, though still relatively undeveloped, gives an opportunity for testing of the hypotheses on delusions against known brain functions and structures. It is hoped that it can be utilised in future in relation to delusional disorder as well as in DMS.

Case No. 15   Delusional misidentification syndrome: Capgras subtype

A previously normal man of 54 was under treatment for arterial hypertension. On several occasions he was noted to have short-lived episodes of confusion, originally diagnosed as 'postural hypotension' due to his antihypertensive medication, but now queried as possible minor strokes. Over a period of several weeks he became very tense and increasingly suspicious, then one day he violently attacked a neighbour, claiming that he was a look-alike impostor who was spying on him. He was very vague as to why such a pretence should be occurring and could not explain how someone was substituted for his neighbour.

He was admitted to a general hospital psychiatric unit where neuroleptics were given with little obvious effect on his irritable behaviour. He was found to be markedly hypertensive and several minor neurological abnormalities were noted, including slight weakness of the left arm. After a medical consultation he was transferred to a general medical unit and a neurological consultation was arranged. Thereafter, he was treated with a new antihypertensive drug and his blood pressure settled. A magnetic resonance investigation (MRI) was carried out and showed a small area of cerebral infarction in the right parieto-temporal area. The neuroleptic was withdrawn and an anticonvulsant was added to his medications. With this, his irritability diminished and after ten days he could talk about his neighbour with no evidence of delusional thinking or anger. When well, he was neuropsychologically tested and was found to have a subtle degree of cognitive disability and of visuospatial impairment, but otherwise functioned normally.

The ultimate diagnosis was that of delusional misidentification syndrome secondary to cerebrovascular disease.

Conclusion

In many ways, primary DMS (i.e. not secondary to another psychiatric disorder) resembles delusional disorder. It is an illness characterized by a delusional system whose content, in this case, involves misidentification. There are several subtypes according to the detailed content of the delusion but overall the form of the illness is similar, no matter the particular nature of the content. The remainder of the personality may be relatively spared but the emotional investment in the delusion is intense and there is associated suspiciousness, anger and, at times, violence. There is no insight in the untreated case. Like delusional disorder, DMS was regarded as rare until recently, but both are now recognized as much more common than was thought. Both disorders have frequently been mistaken in the past for schizophrenia, and have had similar psychodynamic explanations applied to them which have failed to convince. Delusional disorder was excluded from the official diagnostic systems until DSMIIIR reintroduced it in 1987: DMS remains excluded even today.

Treatment of DMS is still somewhat tentative. Authors naturally suggest that the treatment should be appropriate to the underlying disorder if it is schizophrenia or major mood disorder, or should be anticonvulsant medication if it is linked to an organic brain dysfunction. Interestingly, two authors have reported on the successful treatment with pimozide of single cases of Capgras syndrome, one in a 74-year-old woman with a previous history of cerebrovascular accident, and the other in a 67-year-old man with a past history of alcohol abuse (Passer and Warnock, 1991; Tueth and Cheong, 1992). As will be seen in Chapter 13 pimozide is the neuroleptic most often recommended for delusional disorder.

All the above factors suggest a tentative, but reasonably strong, case for including DMS as a distinct disorder within the delusional disorder category. To this writer, the fact that brain investigations in DMS are so much further forward in DMS, as compared with paranoia/delusional disorder, makes it especially exciting, since methods of investigation relevant to one may also be relevant to the other, and inclusion in the same diagnostic category would surely act as an incentive for more scientific exploration of delusional disorder itself. As mentioned in Chapter 8, there are already hints of organic brain abnormalities in elderly patients with delusional disorders, and it is very likely that similar abnormalities will be found in at least some younger individuals with these illnesses.

References

Anderson, D.N. (1988). The delusion of inanimate doubles: implications for understanding the Capgras phenomenon. *Br. J. Psychiat.* **153**:915–917.
Berson, R.J. (1983). Capgras' syndrome. *Am. J. Psychiat.* **140**:969–978.
Brugger, P., Monsch, A.U. and Johnson, S.A. (1996). Repetitive behaviour and repetition avoidance: the role of the right hemisphere. *J. Psychiat. Neurosci.* **21**: 53–56.
Capgras, J. and Reboul-Lachaux, J. (1923). L'illusion des 'sosies' dans un délire systematisé chronique. *Bull. Soc. Clin. Med. Ment.* **2**: 6–16.
Christodoulou, G.N. (1978). Syndrome of subjective doubles. Am. J. Psychiat. **135**: 249–251.
Courbon, P. and Fail, G. (1927). Syndrome d'illusion de Frégoli et schizophrenie. *Bull. Soc. Clin. Med. Ment.* **15**: 121–125.
Courbon, P. and Tusques, J. (1932). Illusion d'intermétamorphose at de charme. *Ann. Med. Psychol.* **90**: 401–405
Cummings, J.L. (1985). Organic delusions: phenomenology, anatomical correlations, and review. *Br. J. Psychiat.* **142**: 184–197.
Debruille, J.B. and Stip, E. (1996). Syndrome de Capgras: évolution des hypothèses. *Can. J. Psychiat.* **41**: 181–187.
Doran, J.M. (1990). The Capgras' syndrome: neurological/neuropsychological perspectives. *Neuropsychology* **4**: 29–42.
Ellis, H.D. (1994). The role of the right hemisphere in the Capgras delusion. *Psychopathology* **27**: 177–185.
Ellis, H.D. and Young, A.W. (1990). Accounting for delusional misidentifications. *Br. J. Psychiat.* **157**: 239–248.
Fishbain, D.A. (1987). The frequency of the Capgras delusions in a psychiatric emergency service. *Psychopathology* **20**:42–47.
Fleminger, S. and Burns, A. (1993). The delusional misidentification syndromes in patients with and without evidence of organic cerebral disorder: a

structured review of case reports. *Biol. Psychiat.* **33**: 22–32.

Förstl, H., Burns, A., Jacoby, R. and Levy, R. (1991). Neuroanatomical correlates of clinical misidentification and misperception in the senile dementia of the Alzheimer type. *J. Clin. Psychiat.* **52**: 268–271.

Gorman, D.G. and Cummings, J.L. (1990). Organic delusional syndrome. *Semin. Neurol.* **10**: 229–238.

Joseph, A.B. (1986). Focal central nervous system abnormalities in patients with misidentification syndromes. *Biblio. Psychiat.* **164**: 69–79.

Landis, T., Cummings, J.L., Benson, D.F. and Palmer, E.P. (1986). Loss of topographic familiarity: an environmental agnosia *Arch. Neurol.* **43**: 132–136.

Manschrek, T.C. (1992). An overview of delusions and delusional disorders: contemporary psychopathology. *Psychiat. Ann.* **22**:229–231.

McAllister, T.W. (1992). Neuropsychiatric aspects of delusions. *Psychiat. Ann.* **22**: 269–277.

Munro, A. (1982). *Delusional Hypochondriasis*. Clarke Institute of Psychiatry Monograph No. 5. Toronto: Clarke Institute of Psychiatry.

Munro, A. (1995). The clasification of delusional disorders. *Psychiat. Clin. N. Am.* **18**: 199–212.

Onuma, T. (1983). Limbic lobe epilepsy with paranoid symptoms: analysis of clinical features and psychological tests. *Folia Psychiat. Neurol. Japon.* **37**:253–258.

Passer, K.M. and Warnock, J.K. (1991). Pimozide in the treatment of Capgras' syndrome. *Psychosomatics* **32**: 446–448.

de Pauw, K.W. (1994a). Delusional misidentification: a plea for an agreed terminology and classification. *Psychopathology* **27**: 123–129.

de Pauw, K.W. (1994b). Psychodynamic approaches to the Capgras delusion: a critical historical review. *Psychopathology* **27**: 154–160.

de Pauw, K.W., Szulecka, T.K. and Poltock, T.L. (1987). Frégoli syndrome after cerebral infarction. *J. Nerv. Ment. Dis.* **175**: 433–438.

Signer, S.F (1994). Localization and lateralization in the delusion of substitution. Capgras syndrome and its variants. *Psychopathology* **27**: 168–176.

Silva, J.A., Sharma, K.K., Leong, G.B. and Weinstock, R. (1992). Dangerousness of the delusional misidentification of children. *J. Forens. Sci., JFSCA* **37**: 830–838.

Spier, S.A. (1992). Capgras' syndrome and the delusions of misidentification. *Psychiat. Ann.* **22**: 279–285.

Tueth, M.J. and Cheong, J.A. (1992). Successful treatment with pimozide of Capgras syndrome in an elderly male. *J. Geriat. Psychiat. Neurol.* **5**: 217–219.

Van Lancker, D.R., Cummings, J.L., Kreiman, J. and Dobkin, B.H. (1988). Phonagnosia: a dissociation between familiar and unfamiliar voices. *Cortex* **24**: 195–209.

Weinstein, E.A. (1994). The classification of delusional misidentification syndromes. *Psychopathology* **27**: 130–135.

10

Folie à deux: an accompaniment of illnesses with delusions

Called 'shared psychotic disorder' in DSMIV and 'induced delusional disorder' in ICD10, this phenomenon occurs when mental symptoms, usually delusions, are communicated from a psychiatrically ill individual to another individual, who accepts them as truth.The two people are nearly always closely associated, especially husband and wife, siblings, or parent–child dyad (Silveira and Seeman, 1995), and social isolation is usually present (Layman and Cohen, 1957; Silveira and Seeman, 1995). The content of shared belief varies from case to case and includes feelings of persecution (Fernando and Frieze, 1985; Kendler and colleagues, 1986; Brooks, 1987), delusional parasitosis (Gieler and Knoll, 1990; Musalek and Kutzer, 1990), conviction of having a child who does not exist (Fishbain, 1987), misidentification of the Capgras type (Hart and McClure, 1989; Ananth, Kaur and Djenderedjian, 1990), and many others. Myers (1988) discusses the phenomenon of shared persecutory beliefs in a cult setting, and refers to Cameron's (1959) description of the 'paranoid pseudocommunity' – the ever-present 'they' who, so far as the patient is concerned, are carrying out the persecution which is not apparent to others.

Folie à deux is not common, but neither is it unduly rare. In 1974, Soni and Rockley reported on 162 cases they had traced up to that time in the English language literature, and Silveira and Seeman (1995) described 123 cases identified from 1942 to 1993. However, one does not find what one is not looking for, and when *folie à deux* is specifically enquired after, it appears to be rather more frequent than is generally thought. For example, the present author found nine occurrences associated with 50 cases suffering from delusional disorder of the somatic subtype (Munro, 1982) and in two instances these were actually *folie à trois*. Musalek and Kutzer (1990) reported a frequency of 8.4 per cent in 107 cases of delusional parasitosis.

It is likely that milder cases are overlooked in general psychiatric practice; also, it is well known that many deluded people resist attending physicians, especially psychiatrists, and in at least one case in this author's own series, the deluded person and the secondary individual colluded to avoid psychiatric assessment.

Enoch and Trethowan (1979) said that 90 per cent of cases occur within families and a number of twin cases have been reported (Nowlin, 1983; Kendler and colleagues, 1986; White, 1995). It seems that the interplay of genetics, close association with an individual who incessantly and vehemently asserts abnormal beliefs, and the effects of social isolation can combine to determine the actual type of *folie à deux* which results.

The modern names given to the condition are open to some degree of semantic criticism. Shared psychotic disorder and induced delusional disorder both imply that the two individuals are psychotic. In many instances that is true of the primary patient, but the recipient of the beliefs is not usually psychotic. In the majority of cases these are impressionable people who adopt untrue beliefs as a result of a long and over-intense association with a deluded person, with social isolation reducing the opportunity for the reality input and reality testing. So, one might say the belief is psychotic but the believer is not.

Another point to be considered is that not all inducers of untrue beliefs are necessarily themselves psychotic. Nearly all cases of *folie à deux* are documented in association with schizophrenia, delusional disorder, severe depressive illness with delusions, or with early dementia, but it is this author's belief that some non-psychotic disorders can also cause *folie à deux*, especially obsessive–compulsive disorder, somatoform disorder and histrionic/dissociative personality disorder. This area is very poorly documented but Kerbeshian (1991) described familial trichotillomania in tandem with obsessive–compulsive disorder.

Gralnick (1942) suggested that there were four subtypes of *folie à deux* as follows:

(1) *Folie imposée*: this is the classical form in which an individual preoccupied with a false belief transmits it to another, impressionable person.

(2) *Folie simultanée*: in this situation there is the simultaneous appearance of identical psychoses in two predisposed people who have usually had a long and very close association. Not uncommonly there is a genetic link and it is claimed that this type is more common in the elderly. As an example, one might find delusional disorders with shared abnormal

beliefs in two unmarried siblings who have become psychotic side by side as the result of living together in isolation for many years. The actual cause of their illness would very likely be determined by shared constitutional factors and the similar clinical features would then be moulded by particular environmental circumstances experienced by both of them.

(3) *Folie communiquée*: there is a transfer of delusions, but only after a long period of resistance by the secondary individual. The delusions are said to persist after separation.

(4) *Folie induite*: new delusions are added to those of a patient under the influence of another deluded patient.

In practice only the first two subtypes need concern us since the last two seem to be variations of *folie imposée*. It is important to differentiate *folie imposée* and *folie simultanée* as will be explained shortly.

Nomenclature

Layman and Cohen (1957) regard *folie à deux* of the *imposée* type not as a separate psychopathological entity but as a 'fortuitous' outcome of certain circumstances, and the present author (Munro, 1986) agrees with this. The primary individual has his own diagnosable illness, whereas the secondary individual has a false belief grafted on to an otherwise relatively normal psyche. So *folie à deux* of this type should be regarded as a phenomenon rather than a disorder in its own right. The terms shared *psychotic disorder* and induced *delusional disorder* are misleading except in *simultanée*-type cases and consideration should be given to changing them. Also, as suggested, the shared belief does not necessarily have to be psychotic or delusional.

Over the years there have been many other descriptive terms for *folie à deux* and Enoch and Trethowan (1979) have cited 'communicated insanity', 'contagious insanity', 'infectious insanity', 'psychosis of association', 'induced psychosis' and 'multiple insanity'. There is also a plethora of terms to describe the pathological relationship, such as 'principle and associate', 'dominant and submissive person', 'patient dyad', etc. The writer has proposed (Munro, 1986), following the suggestion of Enoch and Trethowan, that 'primary patient' and 'secondary patient' is both simple and self-explanatory when discussing *folie imposée*. In *folie simultanée* it is hardly necessary to distinguish primary from secondary.

Treatment

It has to be said that at times it is difficult to distinguish the primary from the secondary patient but, with careful observation, this can usually be accomplished.

In *folie imposée*, the principle method of approach is to treat the primary patient's illness appropriately. It may also help to separate the individuals for a time. With both patients a strong attempt must be made to reduce social isolation and to reintroduce them both to reality. If the primary patient's beliefs recede with treatment (e.g. using a neuroleptic in delusional disorder), the secondary person's beliefs usually also fade and it is rarely appropriate to treat him or her with antipsychotic medication.

On the other hand, if *folie simultanée* is diagnosed, it is usually proper to treat the two patients with neuroleptics or other appropriate medication.

Treatment is theoretically straightforward but in practice can be problematic if the primary patient (or both individuals in *folie simultanée*) is – as is not too uncommon – unco-operative with treatment. In this situation there is often much subterfuge and equal resistance by the secondary patient, so that the psychiatrist may have to expend much time and diplomacy to deal successfully with such a problem. This author has a vivid recollection of a situation where the primary patient was an elderly deluded lady and the secondary patients were her husband and an adult daughter, and all three adamantly refused to accept any psychiatric treatment and formed a solid phalanx against it. This has not been unique in my experience.

A caution to the physician

There is a very important practical point about *folie à deux* to bear in mind. A patient may appear to be deluded, but the physician is perplexed when a close relative strenuously supports the false belief and begins to doubt his or her own judgment. One has seen a number of instances in which much unnecessary physical investigation has occurred in patients with somatic delusions as an outcome of such self-doubt on the physician's part. If one is alert to the possibility of *folie à deux*, a baffling diagnostic problem may become much clearer.

Case No. 16   *Folie à deux*

The index case was a man aged 44 who had had a minor driving accident some eight years previously. He was charged with careless driving, found guilty and given a very minor penalty. Even he agreed at the time that it was an open-or-shut case, but about two years after the hearing he developed the unshakeable conviction that a motor-cycle policeman had given him a misleading signal, thus leading to the accident. He complained so bitterly that an investigation was opened which revealed that no traffic policeman could have been at the scene that day. That only incensed the patient and he brought forward his wife as a witness, who swore that there had been a policeman there and that he had signalled her husband inappropriately. It was only some time later that it was discovered that the wife had actually been in another country visiting relatives at the time.

When faced with this, neither husband nor wife showed any reaction to the contradiction, dealt with it as of no concern and both went on describing what was apparently a delusional memory.

The couple were legally advised to drop their complaint but periodically the husband writes a letter to the authorities or occasionally to the newspapers making exactly the same claim and accusation. After several years he was requested to undergo a psychiatric examination and, in a rather arrogant, offhand manner, he agreed. The interview with husband and wife was totally unsatisfactory as they both refused to give a formal history and spent much of the session asking repetitive questions and raising nitpicking points of order. The wife said nothing of her own accord but echoed and supported everything her husband said.

The best opinion that could be given is that the husband has a delusional disorder, persecutory subtype, with litigious features, and that the wife has a *folie imposée* type of *folie à deux*. No intervention (other than legal, if and when necessary) is possible. Interestingly he continues to work regularly in a minor clerical role in the office of a commercial company.

Conclusion

Be aware of the phenomenon of *folie à deux*. It may not be all that common, but neither is it rare and probably every doctor will find him- or herself misled by an example of it at some time. Being alert to it and being prepared to deal with it using a judicious mixture of tact and firmness may not always work, but it will minimise the chance of physician error in what are usually tricky cases.

References

Ananth, J., Kaur, A. and Djenderedjian, A.H. (1990). Simultaneous folie à deux and Capgras syndrome. *Psychiat. J. Univ. Ottawa* **15**: 41–43.
Brooks, S. (1987). Folie à deux in the aged: variations in psychopathology. *Can. J. Psychiat.* **32**: 61–63.
Cameron, N. (1959). The paranoid pseudocommunity revisited. *Am. J. Sociol.* **65**: 57–61.
Enoch, M.D. and Trethowan, W.H. (1979). *Uncommon Psychiatric Syndromes,* 2nd edn. Bristol: John Wright and Sons.
Fernando, F.P. and Frieze, M. (1985). A relapsing folie à trois. *Br. J. Psychiat.* **146**: 315–324.
Fishbain, D.A. (1987). Folie à deux in the aged. *Can. J. Psychiat.* **32**: 498–499 (letter).
Gieler, U. and Knoll, M. (1990). Delusional parasitosis as 'folie à trois'. *Dermatologica* **181**: 122–125.
Gralnick, A. (1942). Folie à deux: a psychosis of association. A review of 103 cases and the entire English literature. *Psychiat. Quart.* **16**: 230–263.
Hart, J. and McClure, G.M.G. (1989). Capgras' syndrome and folie à deux involving mother and child. *Br. J. Psychiat.* **154**: 552–554.
Kendler, K.S., Robinson, G., McGuire, M. and Spellman, M.P. (1986). Late-onset folie simultanée in a pair of monozygotic twins. *Br. J. Psychiat.* **148**: 463–465.
Kerbeshian, J. (1991). Familial trichotillomania. *Am. J. Psychiat.* **148**: 684 (letter).
Layman, W.A. and Cohen, L. (1957). A modern concept of folie à deux. *J. Nerv. Ment. Dis.* **125**: 412–419.
Munro, A. (1982). *Delusional Hypochondriasis.* Clarke Institute of Psychiatry Monograph No. 5. Toronto: Clarke Institute.
Munro, A. (1986). Folie à deux revisited. *Can. J. Psychiat.* **31**: 233–234.
Musalek, M. and Kutzer, E. (1990). The frequency of shared delusions in delusions of infestation. *Eur. Arch. Psychiat. Neurol. Sci.* **239**: 263–266.
Myers, P.L. (1988). Paranoid pseudocommunity beliefs in a sect milieu. *Soc. Psychiatry Psychiat. Epidemiol.* **23**: 252–255.
Nowlin, N.S. (1983). Anorexia nervosa in twins: case report and review. *J. Clin. Psychiat* **44**: 101–105.
Silveira, J.M. and Seeman, M.V. (1995). Shared psychotic disorder: a critical review of the literature. *Can. J. Psychiat.* **40**: 389–395.
Soni, S.D. and Rockley, G.J. (1974). Socio-clinical substrates of folie à deux. *Br. J. Psychiat.* **125**: 230–235.
White, T.G. (1995). Folie simultanée in monozygotic twins. *Can. J. Psychiat.* **40**: 418–420.

Part IV

Illnesses which are liable to be misdiagnosed as delusional disorders

The wrong way always seems the more reasonable.
George Moore (1852–1933)

Before diagnosis there is the process of differential diagnosis in which the clinician extracts the probable from the possible and the likely from the unlikely. One cannot make a diagnosis without excluding others – no case is ever that black and white.

Since delusional disorder is still an unfamiliar concept to many mental health practitioners we have to alert them to its existence and teach them how to recognize it. We also have to remind them of those other illnesses which may bear some resemblance to it and underline the significant differences between them and it. In Chapter 2, there is mention of several conditions characterized by delusions and the main features which distinguish them from delusional disorder. Here, we wish to amplify some of these distinctions.

This Part comprises two chapters. In Chapter 11, there is a succinct but relatively detailed consideration of two psychotic disorders which are capable at times of being mistaken for delusional disorder, and which are not particularly well-described in the standard literature.

In Chapter 12, which largely consists of case descriptions, the reader's attention is drawn to nonpsychotic illnesses which may superficially resemble delusional disorder. No attempt is made to provide detailed background material here, since this can be obtained from any reputable psychiatric textbook.

11
Reactive and cycloid psychoses: the acute and transient psychotic disorders

Introduction

In this chapter dealing with illnesses which present as psychotic episodes, two separate classes of disorder will be considered. These are:

(1) Brief psychotic disorder (DSMIV) whose counterpart in ICD10 is 'acute and transient psychotic disorder', and which I shall discuss shortly under the heading of 'reactive psychosis'.
(2) Cycloid psychosis, which currently does not have official diagnostic status.

It may be asked why relatively detailed consideration is being given to these two illness types in a book on delusional disorders. The pertinent answer is that, in both illnesses, the acute presentation of a case may be mistaken for some form of delusional disorder, and quite often is.

If brief psychotic disorder and cycloid psychosis were clearly defined and widely accepted entities, a relatively succinct reference to them as differential diagnoses would suffice. Unfortunately, even though the former is described in DSMIV and ICD10, there is a surprising degree of uncertainty about its specific characteristics. The latter diagnosis is simply unfamiliar to many English-speaking psychiatrists, partly because of its absence from official diagnostic schemata. So, in clinical work, one finds much confusion in differentiating between acute and transient psychoses and periodic or cycloid psychoses on the one hand, and distinguishing, on the other hand, between either of these categories and the other major psychotic disorders, including delusional disorders.

As will be described, both the reactive psychoses and the cycloid psychoses are thought to have important constitutional factors in their background, although of markedly different kinds in each case. Brief psychotic disorder (DSMIV), which was 'brief reactive psychosis' in DSMIIIR, is usually thought to be the outcome of a severe stress acting on a constitutional vulnerability, which appears to make sense in the light of the clinical presentation. However, DSMIV also has a sub category in which there are no marked stressors and this surely is a cause for some confusion. It may be that this is an oblique admission by DSMIV that there are two types of episodic psychosis, one precipitated by obvious stress and the other not. If so, it would be much better to admit that this is what is meant and that perhaps the nonstress-related disorder is actually cycloid psychosis, whose features will shortly be described.

In DSMIV, 'brief psychotic disorder' is defined as an illness lasting at least a day but less than a month, which eventually recovers fully. ICD10's 'acute and transient psychotic disorders' show an acute onset of delusions, hallucinations and incomprehensible or incoherent speech, and a maximum of two weeks is stipulated between onset and peak of the disorder. There may also be transient states of perplexity, misidentification or impairment of attention which do not amount to organically caused clouding of consciousness.

Susser and colleagues (1995) generally welcome these descriptions which are an improvement on earlier attempts to describe acute and short-lived psychoses separate from schizophrenia, delusional disorder, schizoaffective disorder and major mood disorder, and with a relatively good prognosis. However, they criticise DSMIV for not distinguishing acute and nonacute varieties and see some of the ICD10 subcategories as unnecessary.

With regard to cycloid psychosis, Perris (1988) pointed out that Kraepelin overlooked this type of mental disorder and, possibly because of this, it has never had a strong representation in classificatory systems based on his work (which includes the current DSM and ICD series). Nevertheless, the concept has persisted in some areas of European and British psychiatry and in recent years there have been mentions in the Canadian (Menuck, Legault and colleagues, 1989) and American (Susser and colleagues, 1995) literatures. In the United Kingdom, Fish (1964) made a seminal contribution to the topic and many of his views still remain pertinent: he was in no doubt that cycloid psychosis was a real and viable diagnostic entity.

So, in the rest of this chapter, an attempt will be made to clarify some difficult issues in relation to the diagnosis of both brief psychotic disorder and cycloid psychosis, with the principal aim of making it easier for the clinician to distinguish them from delusional disorders, and from other functional psychotic illnesses.

Reactive psychoses

A graphic case of confused terminology and conflicting ideologies presents itself in relation to the reactive psychoses. In general, the concept that predominates is that of a psychotic disorder induced by stress which tends to clear up once that stress is removed. Jauch and Carpenter (1988) give a crisp description by calling it a functional psychotic reaction with a good prognosis in which there is a clear relationship with a precipitating stressor. The illness is brief, lasting days to weeks, and there is a return to the previous level of functioning with an absence of chronic residual symptomatology. The onset is an acute one and there is often an 'understandable' preoccupation with the stressful precipitant. Emotional contact with the environment and people in it is retained. These authors also add that 'personality weaknesses' are present.

This is quite similar to the DSMIV category of brief psychotic disorder and is also subsumed within the ICD10 category of acute and transient psychotic disorders. One has to say that the picture is over-simplified in the former and over-elaborated in the latter. DSMIV describes a disturbance of sudden onset with at least one of the following psychotic symptoms: delusions, hallucinations, disorganised speech or grossly disorganised or catatonic behaviour. The duration is at least one day but no more than one month and there is eventual full return to the premorbid level of functioning. An episode may appear following the occurrence of marked stressors or not, or may have its onset in the postpartum period.

DSMIV suggests that pre-existing personality disorders, especially of the paranoid, histrionic, narcissistic, schizotypal or borderline varieties, can predispose to the appearance of the disorder. It says that it is especially common in adolescence and early adulthood and that suicide may be a particular risk. As with other descriptions of the disorder, DSMIV is concerned that it should be carefully differentiated from other psychotic illnesses such as substance-induced or physical illness-induced delirium, schizophreniform disorder, severe mood disorder, or even factitious disorder. There is also an odd footnote stating that some individuals with personality disorders who are under severe stress may have 'brief' (i.e. less than 24 hours) periods of psychotic symptoms. This seems to be stopwatch psychiatry, with an 'over-nice' judgment on the duration of symptoms whose stated duration is already sufficiently arbitrary. Surely if an individual clearly displays the characteristics of a disorder we make the appropriate diagnosis, even if the symptoms are very transient? We do not retreat from doing this in, for example, rapid cycling bipolar mood disorder, so why here?

In any case, we see in DSMIV and ICD10 the description of an illness which is brief, usually related to a combination of external stress and personality vulnerability, and capable of remission when the stress is removed. The overall concept is an acceptable one and most of us who work in the field of acute adult psychiatry are familiar with cases of this sort. However, some unresolved issues remain and these are at least partly due to the disorder's mixed heritage.

Reactive psychosis has been accepted in the past in German and, particularly, Scandinavian psychiatry as a well established and relatively common diagnosis, although even its proponents admit to confusion in its terminology; for example, Retterstøl (1978) mentions reactive psychosis, psychogenic psychosis and constitutional psychosis as synonyms, Noreik (1970) talks of reactive paranoid psychosis, and Jørgensen and Jensen (1988) discuss reactive delusional psychosis. In most of the descriptions a longer duration (even up to two years) than is accepted by DSMIV and ICD10 is usual. Dahl (1987) is particularly critical of over-use of the concept of reactive psychosis and proposes that it must be restricted to functional psychoses which are not schizophrenia, delusional disorder, or major mood disorder.

This stricture is necessary since, as we all know, features of the early stages of a psychotic illness may be so indiscriminate that we cannot at that point decide the exact nature of the diagnosis. A positive family history and a significant previous history may be helpful but are not pathognomonic. A temptation to make a diagnosis of reactive psychosis is that one is then implying a severe psychiatric illness but is also suggesting a good prognosis until proven otherwise. That is a charitable, but not particularly incisive, approach. A number of authors (Faergeman, 1963; Noreik, 1970; McCabe and Strömgren, 1975; Jauch and Carpenter, 1988; Jørgensen and Jensen, 1988) have shown that at follow-up a high proportion of apparent reactive psychosis cases have actually evolved into schizophrenic or major mood disorders. Jauch and Carpenter (1988) make particular comment on the difficulties raised by diagnostic variation, which of course can arise both at the time of the episode's onset and at the time of follow-up assessment. McCabe (1976) says that schizophrenia with good prognosis is not uncommonly really reactive psychosis. However, it must also be noted that a substantial number of cases (50 per cent in Jauch and Carpenter's estimate) do not become chronically psychotic and some of these may show repeated episodes of stress-induced, remitting psychosis, especially if they continue to experience marked ongoing stresses.

Another line of descent for the current diagnosis of reactive psychosis is from the concept known in the past as hysterical psychosis. This diagnosis was fairly popular in English-language psychiatry until the 1970s, but is now rarely referred to. Its description is similar in many ways to that of reactive psychosis but with a heavier emphasis on the putative personality and psychodynamic factors which were thought to be of predisposing significance. A source article is that by Hirsch and Hollender (1969), and Martin (1971) outlined the psychodynamics as they were understood at that time.

Cavenar, Sullivan and Maltbie (1979) describe hysterical psychosis in similar terms to reactive psychosis, as an illness which usually has a sudden, dramatic onset with hallucinations (often of a visual kind), delusions, derealisation, depersonalisation and bizarre behaviour. There is no schizophrenic looseness of associations and affect is neither flat nor blunted. The duration is hours to weeks and there are no residual effects. It is said to occur most often in females with hysterical personalities who react to an affect-laden situation by becoming distraught and displaying a breakdown of personality integration. This occurs after an extremely distressing event such as an unwanted sexual advance and the authors quote Brill (see Hollender and Hirsch, 1964) as saying that it is 'more like the simple distortions of reality of a very angry or fearful child, which disappear when emotional control is achieved'.

In DSMIII (1980) there was a section on brief reactive psychosis which was very bald and described 'Psychotic symptoms immediately following a recognizable psychosocial stressor that would evoke significant symptoms of distress in almost anyone'. The duration was a few hours to two weeks. There was no mention of personality factors. In addition, DSMIII described acute paranoid disorder, an illness of less than six months' duration, usually of sudden onset and rarely becoming chronic. This condition was said to be seen most commonly in individuals who had experienced drastic environmental change, such as immigrants, refugees, prisoners of war, inductees into military service or people leaving home for the first time. What is not mentioned specifically is that many of these people also had marked persecutory ideas, so in the habit of the time were likely to be diagnosed as having a paranoid illness on that account.

By the time of DSMIIIR it was felt that these two categories overlapped significantly and acute paranoid disorder was dropped. The description of brief reactive psychosis was expanded somewhat to indicate symptoms similar to those mentioned in reference to hysterical psychosis (see above).

Duration was now allowed to be from a few hours up to one month and restitution to premorbid functioning was usual. Pre-existing personality disorder might predispose to the illness. The subsequent DSMIV and ICD10 descriptions are not dissimilar.

We therefore have an illness, the premises of which are widely accepted but whose details remain vague. In particular the duration is in dispute: the lower limit can probably be as brief as a few hours and the upper limit is one month (DSMIV) or, alternatively, a considerable number of months according to various Scandinavian authors. (The longer the upper limit the more danger there seems to be of including cases of other mental disorders.) There is an interplay of stress factors and personality instability, the proportions of which are probably unique to each individual, and there is general agreement that the episode usually clears up when the stress clears up.

But what do we make of DSMIVs brief psychotic disorder *without* marked stressors which was mentioned previously (see p.196). At this point, the best that one can suggest is that either it means that the stressor is presumed to be present but cannot be detected (which is unsatisfactory), or that a rather different condition is being described, perhaps a cycloid psychosis, if only that diagnosis were more accepted in the English-speaking world.

And finally, in the context of the present volume, brief psychotic disorder has to be emphasized once again as a condition which, in its florid presentation and with its frequent content of delusions, often of a persecutory nature, but with its retention of strong affective elements, may readily be mistaken for a delusional disorder if only the cross-sectional picture is taken into account. The confusion is more likely to be with paraphrenia/paranoid schizophrenia than with paranoia/delusional disorder, but this writer has certainly seen errors towards either of these diagnostic areas being made on a number of occasions.

Case No. 17   Brief psychotic disorder

A woman of 34, of Afro-Caribbean background, was admitted to an acute psychiatric inpatient unit for observation, having been brought by relatives to the hospital. Because the patient could not give a history at the time they reported that, for the past 48 hours, she had become increasingly distraught, restless and irrational. She had not slept for two nights, was extremely agitated, said she had visions of her dead grandmother and heard the voices of God and of Satan telling her she was to be devoured alive.

Her family said she was a single mother with two young children and she lived with her parents. She was normally cheerful and moderately outgoing as well as being conscientious and a good mother. She worried a lot about financial matters and, at times, could become distressed when money was short. She had become increasingly anxious recently because she had been put on reduced hours at work and there was a danger of redundancy. Just before the onset of the present symptoms she had been badly frightened when her younger son disappeared for several hours, and she was not relieved when he turned up with an innocent explanation. The symptoms of distress then rapidly escalated on their own. She had never had an illness like this before, and there was no history of significant alcohol or drug abuse. The family denied any mental illness in relatives.

In hospital she was extremely restless, appeared confused and disoriented, behaved in unusual ways, for example hiding under her bed to avoid Satan, trying to put her head under water to stop the voices reaching her ears and running, naked and screaming, through the unit. She appeared profoundly over-alerted, with exaggeration of autonomic responses. Despite the apparently psychotic picture, she showed some appropriate affective responses, in particular appearing almost normally happy when her children were allowed to visit her briefly.

After observing and treating her with anti-anxiety agents, a tentative diagnosis of brief psychotic disorder was made. The patient slept for 14 hours with sedation and awoke much calmer, normally oriented and apparently in clear consciousness. She still talked a good deal about God and the Devil, but 24 hours later no longer appeared distressed by her thoughts. After four days in hospital she was discharged home and reported that she felt normal at that time. She herself had no explanation for the episode other than to say, 'I was worried at the time'.

Cycloid psychosis (also known as periodic psychosis)

Fish (1964) succinctly encapsulated this as an illness characterized by schizophrenic symptoms and a manic-depressive course. Much of the writing on the subject is German. Kleist (1928) described a widespread group of disorders with intermittent features which he named 'the phasophrenias', which included bipolar and unipolar mood disorders and various types of delusional illnesses and hallucinoses. Leonhard refined certain aspects of this classification and went on to delineate three psychoses which he grouped together as 'cycloid' (a term he borrowed from Kleist) because they recurred like mood disorders. He also described them as having bipolar features since opposite symptoms would occur at different phases of the illness. (This use of the term 'bipolar' should not be confused with its modern connotation of bipolar mood disorder.)

Leonhard (1961) describes these three psychoses as 'motility psychosis' (hyperkinetic–akinetic), 'confusion psychosis' (excited–inhibited), and 'anxiety-elation psychosis' (angst–elation). However, he admits that the features of the three often overlap and intermingle: modern workers who diagnose cycloid psychosis recognize the existence of the symptom clusters but usually do not try to differentiate them as separate disorders. Leonhard insisted that the overall group of cycloid psychoses was separate from major mood disorder, schizophrenia or delusional disorder, and that the diagnosis should be made by a combination of cross-sectional and longitudinal observations of the case. The present author agrees with that viewpoint.

Clinical features

These have been best defined by Perris (1988) and Cutting (1990). The illness is particularly characterized by:

(1) The presence of a psychotic state (i.e. the patient is out of touch with reality).
(2) Mood swings during the psychotic state which are usually rapid and frequent, with sudden elation, depression and severe anxiety, sometimes interspersed with periods of relative normality. Symptoms are polymorphous and shifting.
(3) At least two of the following: (*a*) paranoia-like symptoms (i.e. mainly mood-incongruent delusions or hallucinations); (*b*) motility disturbance, usually an acceleration or slowing of movement but not catatonia; (*c*) confusion, anywhere between mild perplexity and severe disorientation, and often fluctuating in degree; (*d*) pananxiety, which Cutting translates as 'angst',meaning extreme fear of imminent disaster or death; (*e*) ecstasy, which is much more intense than simple elation (and which appears to be the least common of this group of symptoms).

(4) Complete resolution of symptoms after the episode, usually within weeks or months but sometimes after a much longer time.

In addition, the illness has a marked tendency to recur and each episode in a given individual tends to resemble the foregoing episodes closely.

Precipitating factors

It seems to be generally agreed that the majority of episodes occur spontaneously (Perris, 1988; Cutting, 1990), although there may be apparent precipitating factors in a relatively small number of cases. However, a significant minority arise in the postpartum period.

Genetic factors

Cutting (1990) points out that, since the diagnosis of cycloid psychosis in an index case is often dubious, the diagnosis of mental illness in the relatives may be even more so. However, Leonhard (1961) claimed that the disorder bred true in the families of 40 per cent of his cases, and Fish also describes a family pattern for the illness. Perris (1988) believed that his cases show an excess of similar disorders in close relatives, but he sounds a note of caution citing, as does Cutting, the relative lack of scientific precision in the family studies carried out to date.

Course and prognosis

The typical case of cycloid psychosis starts acutely with few or no prodromal symptoms, rapidly reaches its peak (usually within a few days) and resolves equally quickly with complete recovery in a few weeks or months, although the length of an individual episode is highly variable. The prognosis of the individual episode is good (Perris and Brockington, 1981) and only a few patients seem to be left with mild residual symptoms (Perris, 1988).

There is a high frequency of relapse and, for example, Leonhard reports cases with 30 or more episodes. Attacks can come in clusters, then be separated by long intervals of freedom in the same patient. Occasionally, episodes can appear increasingly frequently until the patient is almost continuously ill. Some older studies suggested that almost 50 per cent of patients eventually show complete remission.

Leonhard (1980) warned that many cases of cycloid psychosis are iatrogenically kept in a toxic state when the doctor makes a misdiagnosis and maintains the patient inappropriately on a psychotropic medication.

Other characteristics

A very high proportion of cases apparently occur in women, even higher than can be accounted for by the puerperal factor. There is a wide range of age of onset in both sexes, with Cutting (1990) quoting a mean age of 31.5 years for his series.

Treatment

There has long been a consensus that cycloid psychosis best responds to antidepressant treatment and Perris (1988) reports benefit from electroconvulsive therapy (six to eight treatments), with haloperidol in the acute phase, and lithium as a preventive measure. On the other hand, well designed treatment studies are lacking and in an illness whose episodes are self-limiting it is always going to be difficult to know if it improved spontaneously or because of a recently-administered medication.

Diagnostic issues

Most authors who write on the topic of cycloid psychosis see it as an entity but there are some (e.g. Cutting, 1990) who contend that it is a variant of bipolar mood disorder. However, as Perris (1988) points out, it is most often misdiagnosed as schizophrenia or schizoaffective disorder and, in the present author's experience, there has been contact with a number of cases wrongly diagnosed as delusional disorder. If one takes a purely cross-sectional view of the illness it usually shows schizophrenia-like features most prominently, but with a considerable loading of mood symptoms and, at times, within the episode intervals of apparent normality. If the acute and episodic nature of the illness is not appreciated, the well-retained affect and the seeming movement between psychosis and a symptom-free state may well suggest paraphrenia or paranoia/delusional disorder.

Case No. 18   Cycloid psychosis

A 62-year-old widow broke her ankle and had the fracture reduced under anaesthetic. Within 24 hours of the operation she became agitated, confused and deluded. For the next three weeks, while living with a son and his family, her behaviour became increasingly bizarre, including posturing, rolling on the floor, shouting and screaming, urinating and defaecating in public and saying that her deceased husband was tormenting her. She appeared to be auditorily hallucinated.

She was admitted to a psychiatric unit where she was found to be disoriented to place and person but not to time. Despite being deluded and hallucinated and behaving in an erratic, irrational manner, she had warm affect and, in brief conversations, could show superficially normal emotional responses. From her previous records and from interviews with her three adult children it was learned that she had been having episodes like this since the age of 16. Although the history was not altogether clear, it seemed that each episode had a markedly 'punched-out' quality, with rapid onset and resolution. The duration of an episode varied between four and ten weeks. On previous admissions, varying diagnoses had been made, such as schizophrenia, paranoia, organic brain disorder, schizoaffective disorder and atypical bipolar mood disorder. Recovery was apparently complete between episodes and until this occasion, the patient had been well for approximately 15 years. Four years ago she had coped adequately with the death of her husband. Her family said that, although a quiet person who now lived alone, she had always been emotionally warm, a good wife and mother and someone who, apart from her periods of illness, lived a very normal existence. The only positive family history of psychiatric illness was in a maternal aunt who had been diagnosed as schizophrenic, but no details were available.

After observation a diagnosis of cycloid psychosis was made and, since the consensus about treatment seems to be that this should be treated as an atypical bipolar illness, she was prescribed a combination of valproic acid and perphenazine. She improved moderately on this and was no longer confused or disoriented but remained hallucinated and deluded. After four weeks of treatment she suddenly began to be brighter, more active and more realistically concerned about hygiene, her broken ankle, and her outside affairs. Two weekend passes to stay with family confirmed the improvement and she was discharged to her son's home to convalesce.

The family commented that she was now fully back to her normal self. The patient appeared to have very little recollection of her illness or of the previous episodes although she had good insight and accepted that she had a recurrent mental disorder. She was referred for outpatient follow-up and was asked to continue taking the valproate and a small dose of neuroleptic, although there was doubt that her medications actually had anything to do with her recovery.

Bouffée délirante

Before finishing this chapter and for completeness' sake, mention should be made of this related diagnostic concept, which continues to be used in Francophone psychiatry (Allodi, 1982).

Bouffée délirante is the present-day remnant of a much larger concept from late nineteenth century French psychiatry, originally proposed by Magnan (1893). In relatively modern times it was divided into reactive *bouffée délirante* (similar to acute reactive psychosis in DSMIIIR) and *bouffée délirante*, Magnan type, which is essentially cycloid psychosis (Perris, 1988). Not all French-speaking psychiatrists clearly differentiate between these two forms.

Nowadays (Pichot, 1986) it is most often described as a remitting paranoid psychosis with florid but variable delusions; a mixture of unstable mood, illusions, hallucinations, and clouded consciousness. The onset is sudden and there is rapid recovery within days or weeks, but recurrence is not infrequent. If there is not full recovery between episodes, a diagnosis of schizophrenia or delusional disorder is considered, but within the acute episode the features may resemble delusional disorder. External precipitating factors are usually absent.

Superficially, it seems that the modern usage is closer to that of a brief reactive psychosis/brief psychotic disorder but the English-language literature is unhelpful in rendering the concept clearer: for example, Sim (1988) simply refers to it as an acute delusional state. Gelder and colleagues (1996) say that the ICD10 category of acute and transient psychotic disorder regards *bouffée délirante* and cycloid psychosis as synonymous. This book is not the place to enter into the finer points of a debate on this subject, but is certainly a vehicle for expressing dismay once more at the dreadful confusion in semantics that still pervades so much of psychiatry.

Conclusion

Transient or remitting psychoses, separate from delusional disorder, schizophrenia or major mood disorder, do exist. As presently conceived they are a mixed group, but are capable of being divided into two major categories, the 'reactive' (brief psychotic disorder minus the subcategory of 'without marked stressors') and the 'cycloid'. Doubtless, there are other 'residual', 'atypical' illnesses which could be included in the category but it is vital that psychiatrists should clarify their thinking on these two main subcategories and be able to diagnose either with confidence. As already noted, examples of either of them may temporarily resemble delusional disorders. Knowledge of their features will prevent any serious or embarrassing diagnostic mistakes being made.

References

Allodi, F. (1982). Acute paranoid reaction (bouffée délirante) in Canada. *Can. J. Psychiat.* **27**: 366–373.

Brill, N.Q., cited in Hollender, M.H. and Hirsch, S.J. (1964). Hysterical psychosis. *Am. J. Psychiat* **120**: 1066–1074.

Cavenar, J.O., Sullivan, J.L. and Maltbie, A.A. (1979). A clinical note on hysterical psychosis. *Am. J. Psychiat.* **136**: 830–832.

Cutting, J. (1990). Relationship between cycloid psychosis and typical affective psychosis. *Psychopathology* **23**: 212–219.

Dahl, A.A. (1987). Problems concerning the concept of reactive psychoses. *Psychopathology* **20**: 79–86.

Diagnostic and Statistical Manual of Mental Disorders, 3rd edn (DSMIII) (1980). Washington, DC: American Psychiatric Association.

Diagnostic and Statistical Manual of Mental Disorders, 3rd edn revised (DSMIIIR) (1987). Washington, DC: American Psychiatric Association.

Diagnostic and Statistical Manual of Mental Disorders, 4th edn (DSMIV) (1994). Washington, DC: American Psychiatric Association.

Faergeman, P.M. (1963). *Psychogenic Psychoses*. London: Butterworth.

Fish, F. (1964). The cycloid psychoses. *Comp. Psychiat.* **5**: 155–169.

Gelder, M., Gath, D., Mayou, R. and Cowen, P. (1996). *Oxford Textbook of Psychiatry*, p. 261. Oxford: Oxford University Press.

Hirsch, S.J. and Hollender, M.H. (1969). Hysterical psychosis: clarification of the concept. *Am. J. Psychiat.* **125**: 81–87.

International Statistical Classification of Diseases, 10th edn (ICD10) 1992–3 Geneva: World Health Organization.

Jauch, D.A. and Carpenter, W.T. (1988). Reactive psychosis I: Does the pre-DSMIII concept define a third psychosis? *J. Nerv. Ment. Dis.* **176**: 72–81.

Jørgensen, P. and Jensen, J. (1988). An attempt to operationalize reactive delusional psychosis. *Acta Psychiat. Scand.* **78**: 627–631.

Kleist, K. (1928). Über zykloide, paranoide und epileptoide Psychosen und über die Frage der Degenerationspsychosen. *Schweiz Arch. Neurol. Psychiat.* **23**: 1–17.

Leonhard, K. (1961). Cycloid psychoses – endogenous psychoses which are neither schizophrenic nor manic-depressive. *J. Ment. Sci.* **107**: 633–648.

Leonhard, K. (1980). *Aufteilung der endogenen Psychosen*, 5th edn. Jena: Akademie Verlag.

Magnan, V. (1893) *Leçons Cliniques sur les Maladies Mentales*, 2nd edn. Paris: Bataille.

Martin, P.A. (1971). Dynamic considerations of the hysterical psychosis. *Am. J. Psychiat.* **128**: 101–104.

McCabe, M.S. (1976). Reactive psychoses and schizophrenia with good prognosis. *Arch. Gen. Psychiat.* **33**: 571–576.

McCabe, M.S. and Strömgren, E. (1975). Reactive psychoses: a family study. *Arch. Gen. Psychiat.* **32**: 447–454.

Menuck, M., Legault, S., Schmidt, P. and Remington, G. (1989). The nosologic status of the remitting atypical psychoses. *Comp. Psychiat.* **30**: 53–73.

Noreik, K. (1970). *Followup and Classification of Functional Psychoses with Special Reference to Reactive Psychoses.* Oslo: Universitetsforlaget.

Perris, C. (1988). The concept of cycloid psychotic disorder. *Psychiat. Dev.* **1**: 37–56.

Perris, C. and Brockington, I.F. (1981). Cycloid psychoses and their relation to the major psychoses. In *Biological Psychiatry*, ed. C. Perris, pp. 447–450. Amsterdam: Elsevier.

Pichot, P. (1986). The concept of 'bouffée délirante' with special reference to the Scandinavian concept of reactive psychoses. *Psychopathology* **19**: 35–43.

Retterstøl, N. (1978). The Scandinavian concept of reactive psychosis, schizophreniform psychosis and schizophrenia. *Psychiat. Clin. (Basel)* **11**: 180–187.

Sim, A. (1988). *Symptoms in the Mind. An Introduction to Descriptive Psychopathology*, p. 313. London: Baillière Tindall.

Susser, E., Fennig, P.H.S., Jandorf, L., Amador, X. and Bromet, E. (1995). Epidemiology, diagnosis and course of brief psychoses. *Am. J. Psychiat.* **152**: 1743–1748.

12
Non-psychotic disorders which may simulate delusional disorders

.

The 'group A' (paranoid, schizoid and schizotypal) personality disorders

Not only do Group A personality disorders have to be differentiated from the delusional disorders, but it has already been noted in Chapter 7 that they may be on a continuum ('the paranoid spectrum') with these disorders. This may involve consideration of premorbid personality patterns in delusional disorder patients, as well as abnormalities of personality in the close relatives of patients with schizophrenia and related disorders. Kendler and Gruenberg (1982) found that paranoid personality disorder was relatively frequent in the families of individuals with 'schizophrenic spectrum' conditions (which would include delusional disorder). Kendler and colleagues (1984) noted that schizophrenia-related personality disorders were more common in the first degree relatives of schizophrenics compared with those of normal controls. The present author (Munro, 1982) reported that 28 per cent of a group of 50 delusional disorder, somatic subtype, cases were regarded as having longstanding personality disorders, mostly of a schizoid type. Thirty per cent of the same group described psychiatric problems in close relatives, mostly related to personality factors or alcohol abuse, but with no further details. Winokur (1985) found that the close relatives of 29 nonhallucinating delusional disorder patients showed an excess of suspicious, secretive or jealous personality features and, in a proportion of cases, actual delusions.

However, Dorfman, Shields and Delisi (1993) reported that although they found many types of personality disorder in the near relatives of a group of schizophrenics, paranoid personality disorder was no more common than in the relatives of normal controls. Fulton and Winokur (1993), looking at individuals with schizoid personality disorder, found no excess of schizophrenia in their families compared with controls.

Here, we shall limit our considerations to examples of cases which bear sufficient resemblance to a delusional disorder as to require diagnostic differentiation.

Case No. 19 Paranoid personality disorder

This patient is a business executive aged 39. Although reasonably successful in his career, he remains unfulfilled and unhappy with his progress. He married at the age of 29 but divorced five years later. He blames his ex-wife for the break-up, but in psychotherapy he has described his attitudes towards her in terms of being over-demanding, jealous, and perpetually dissatisfied, while always maintaining a self-justifying stance.

He works hard but gives the impression of being unimaginative. He strongly resents younger individuals gaining more rapid promotion and believes that his superiors are keeping him back because he is a potential threat to them. On a number of occasions he has complained about them to the company directors and does not see that this might make him unpopular or brand him as a troublemaker. His general attitude is rigid and quasi-puritanical: if he causes trouble because he is displeased he rationalises this by saying that he has found that his bosses are inefficient and corrupt.

His social life is limited and he has no close friends. His only outside interest is his membership of a local dramatic society. He says he enjoys this but believes he has been prevented from being the male lead on more than one occasion because he is 'not one of the clique'. He visits his elderly parents from time to time but does not communicate with other family members, with whom he has fallen out, one by one.

At this time he has come for psychotherapy complaining of pervasive anxiety feelings. He is also afraid that his alcohol consumption is rising although the amounts he quotes do not seem alarming. He reports that he has had several other attempts at psychotherapy or counselling in the past but gave up because none of the therapists were 'intellectually capable and were not interested in dealing with his needs'. After three outpatient sessions this time, he has twice been late for appointments, has tried to provoke an argument, and has attempted to get the therapist to join in his criticism of a professional colleague who was one of his previous therapists. The patient has already said that he is not happy with progress and will give the present psychiatrist 'one more try'.

Case No. 20   Schizoid personality disorder

This lady was never a psychiatric patient but was an acquaintance of the author. She was unmarried and had been left a certain amount of money by elderly parents when they died. She continued to live in the family house by herself and paid little attention to its maintenance, so that it was becoming shabby and rundown. An only child, she had no friends of her own but a few people who had known her parents kept some contact with her. She never initiated any meetings but seemed quite pleased when someone called on her, although visits always had to be arranged well beforehand.

She belonged to a church and attended regularly but took no part in its wider activities. She never seemed to buy new clothes so her appearance became increasingly old-fashioned, but she had no obvious eccentricities of behaviour. She always avoided people when possible and if spoken to in the street she would smile, mutter a few words and pass on. At home she led a very uneventful life, doing some sewing, looking after three cats, listening to radio (she would never buy a television set), and going out for solitary walks, usually in the twilight.

When visited she was welcoming, apparently unaware of the dustiness of her surroundings, and could conduct a conversation with a certain quiet humour. She was fond of reminiscing but never allowed visits to last more than an hour. She was never heard to say anything which could be regarded as bizarre or indicative of any mental illness.

She developed cancer of the breast and only consulted her family physician when it was well advanced. Her attitude to the illness was passive and fatalistic and she rejected offers of help by acquaintances. She seemed to be fully aware that her condition was fatal. She attended church as long as she was able then quietly entered a nursing home, using her funds to ensure she had a single room. She died quite peacefully at the age of 45 and despite her solitariness several staff members in the home commented that she had been a very nice woman.

Case No. 21   Schizotypal personality disorder

A woman aged 36, but looking considerably younger, has been admitted to an inpatient psychiatric unit on several occasions having taken overdoses of analgesics. After recovery she invariably denies having had any suicidal intent but whether this is true or not is very unclear.

As a child she was noted to be solitary and her school performance was erratic. She left school at the age of 17 and became involved with the local drug culture. She is vague about specifics but was certainly a heavy user of marijuana and LSD. It seems likely that she also experimented for a time with opioids and intermittently with cocaine. Her existence has been a drifting one. At times she lives in communes and at other times she sets up in her own accommodation, in and out of which other people seem to move casually. She admits to numerous sexual liaisons, mostly with males but occasionally with females, and she has had several venereal infections over the years, fortunately never syphilis nor AIDS to this point.

The patient has difficulty in providing a history. Her conversation is diffuse, circumstantial and nongoal-directed. She mostly answers by analogy and often makes references to esoteric topics which she assumes the listener will understand. At various times she has been involved with fringe therapy groups, pseudo-philosophical movements and a number of cults. She believes in the supernatural and communicates with gods from several ancient religions. Although she says she hears voices, when this is pursued she says they are 'inner voices' and they do not appear to be hallucinations. She is oriented and there is never any clouding of consciousness. Her appearance and clothing are somewhat odd but probably in keeping with her cultural background.

Mood is often dysphoric. She can never explain her overdoses but it is suspected that they usually occur in the withdrawal phase following heavy drug use. When she recovers she is never willing to confide in hospital staff, refuses outpatient follow-up and is lost to view until the next incident occurs, usually two or three years later.

At no time has she ever been noted to have a frank psychotic breakdown.

Conclusion

Group A personality disorders are not in themselves delusional disorders nor schizophrenic illnesses but, on occasion, may be precursors of these conditions. Careful diagnostic skills are needed so as not mistakenly to label the personality disorder as a psychosis, but also to ensure that a psychotic disorder emerging insidiously from one of them is not overlooked.

Incidentally, the diagnosis of borderline personality disorder is a popular one in North America. Conventionally, it is included in the 'group B' personality disorders (along with antisocial personality disorder) but case descriptions often make it seem more or less indistinguishable from paranoid personality disorder. This author knows of no work relating borderline personality disorder to the genesis of delusional disorder, but it seems not unlikely that the thought may have occurred to someone.

Obsessive–compulsive disorders

Case No. 22   Obsessive–compulsive disorder (with bizarre features)

The patient was a 48-year-old unmarried woman who owned a highly patronised business in a small town and who was a prominent member of the church and the community. She was regarded as a somewhat secretive person with no close friends but otherwise appeared generally warm and friendly. In all her activities she was recognized to be very organised and precise. Her health was usually good but after a severe attack of influenza she was admitted to hospital with pneumonia. Her sister came from another city to help and, without the patient's permission, gained entry to her house, which she had never visited before.

To her amazement she found that only the kitchen and bathroom were habitable. Every other part of the house was crammed with objects – furniture, radios, appliances, cans of food, etc. – often many of each. The staircase was stacked with neatly packed bundles of newspapers and magazines, and tied-up piles of documents filled every other conceivable space.

She tackled the patient about her house when she had recovered from her pneumonia and the latter was at first furious that her sister had intruded, then distressed and ashamed. She refused to explain the state of her home and told her sister angrily to mind her own business, that she had bought everything in the house and did not want anything changed. Following discharge from hospital she agreed to see her family physician who had been told by the sister of the situation. She was almost as uncommunicative with him but he was convinced after the interview that she was not in any way psychotic. She refused to see a specialist, but the family physician discussed the case with a psychiatrist, while maintaining the patient's confidence. The possibility of an obsessive–compulsive disorder or of a delusional disorder was considered, with the former being the more likely.

The patient declined any treatment and after her physical health recovered she resumed her business and church activities. She would occasionally visit the family doctor for incidental health matters but her hoarding behaviour was never alluded to. Several years later she was maintaining her high-profile position in the community with no external evidence of mental illness.

Somatoform disorders, with especial emphasis on body dysmorphic disorder

The category of somatoform disorders is a poorly researched one. Until recently it was also one which promised poor results in terms of psychiatric intervention (Lloyd, 1986). Nowadays, the picture has improved considerably since the introduction of treatment with serotonergic antidepressants. This treatment approach, often linked with cognitive–behavioural therapy, has been shown to produce good results in cases of body dysmorphic disorder (Phillips and colleagues, 1993; Rosen, 1995), and there are scattered reports of improvement with similar treatment of other somatoform disorders.

Some workers (for example, McElroy, Phillips, Keck, Hudson and Pope, 1993) have proposed that nondelusional and delusional forms of dysmorphic belief lie on the same spectrum and that cases of nondelusional hypochondriasis may sometimes decompensate to episodes of psychosis with delusions. These episodes have been equated with delusional disorder of the somatic subtype (Phillips and McElroy, 1993).

However, delusional disorder is not an episodic illness and there is no evidence at present of consistent premorbid obsessive–compulsive features in the personalities of sufferers. In addition, the cases described by the above authors do not respond well to neuroleptics but do improve with selective serotonin reuptake inhibitor (SSRI) antidepressants. The present author does not find a convincing link between such cases and cases of delusional disorder, and instead regards them as falling into the category of brief psychotic disorder (with marked stressor, in DSMIV terms), the stressor being the illness itself and the severe anxiety often associated with it.

Nevertheless, this is an area worthy of more research and, at the very least, one may say that somatoform disorder, especially body dysmorphic disorder, must be considered and excluded before delusional disorder, somatic subtype, is diagnosed.

The following case illustrates the apparent resemblances between body dysmorphic disorder and delusional disorder with dysmorphic beliefs.

Case No. 23   Body dysmorphic disorder

An attractive 35-year-old single mother of three children was referred for psychiatric opinion by her family physician. The patient was extremely anxious and insisted that she was physically disgusting because of abdominal striae related to her three pregnancies. She had made repeated demands for cosmetic surgery over the previous two years, was furious at being denied this, and was initially resistant to psychiatric assessment. Finally she agreed because it had been suggested that the psychiatrist might recommend surgery on 'mental health grounds'.

At initial interview she was agitated, dejected, angry and demanding. She was not interested in any psychodynamic investigation of her symptoms. However, following a fairly lengthy session it seemed reasonably certain that she was not deluded, she could be engaged in debate about her symptoms and she could even agree they might seem unreasonable to others. She did not claim that other people could see the striae when she was clothed but claimed that the marks kept her from normal activities such as swimming, and ruined her chance of ever remarrying. She said she would kill herself if she could not have reparative surgery and, at first, refused to accept psychotropic medication.

She declined to return to see the psychiatrist but fortunately had trust in the family doctor who, on advice, eventually persuaded her to accept an SSRI antidepressant. Her compliance was poor at first but when she got some relief from anxiety she reluctantly agreed to take the medication in adequate dosage. Despite grumbling about side effects (which were not severe) she began to improve. Distress and preoccupation were diminished, although they did not totally disappear. After two years the patient, although still chronically disgruntled, was involved in paid work, had some degree of social activity and said, 'There's no point in trying to get plastic surgery because I'll never be able to afford it'.

Dissociative disorder

Case No. 24   Dissociative disorder

A 38-year-old woman of borderline intelligence has been admitted to inpatient psychiatric services at least 30 times since her late teens. Early admissions record 'hallucinations', 'delusions', 'poverty of thought' and 'bizarre behaviours'. She was treated with neuroleptics but results were poor and she lived a marginal existence in the community with repeated breakdowns and psychiatric admissions. In the mid-1980s, apparently because of lack of deterioration in her symptoms she was re-diagnosed from chronic schizophrenia to delusional disorder. Her condition got no better as a result of this or from continued neuroleptic treatment.

At a time when there was a flush of enthusiasm for the diagnosis of multiple personality disorder she was re-assessed and declared to be suffering from this. Her 'hallucinations' were said to be the voices of her alternative personalities, memory blanks were the result of intermittent takeover by these alternatives, strange behaviours were due to the acting out of more childish selves, and thought disorder was seen to be due to numerous intrusions of other personalities' thinking. Given this diagnosis and a highly permissive approach to treatment, the patient became blatantly disturbed in her behaviour, with a great deal of acting out and a number of dramatic but ineffectual suicide attempts. She was encouraged by her therapists to blame all of this on early-life sexual abuse (which probably had occurred) and the 'needs' of her alternative personalities. All medication was discouraged except anti-anxiety drugs and she became habituated to one of the benzodiazepines.

After several years of increasingly chaotic lifestyle, the patient was once more re-assessed. It was agreed that she had neither schizophrenia nor delusional disorder, but was of lower intelligence and had severe personality disorder with marked dependent and histrionic features. It was also agreed that she had a dissociative disorder but not a multiple personality disorder.

Recent treatment has largely consisted of closer supervision in the community with essentially practical support and recognition that this patient's dependency can be helped but not eliminated. Psychological approaches include firm but kindly handling, simplified cognitive therapy and very concrete behavioural methods, mainly to counter stress and anxiety. Groups for anger management and anxiety control are available and the patient attends from time to time.

She has not been on antipsychotic medication for several years and shows absolutely no evidence of delusional disorder or schizophrenia.

Factitious disorder

Case No. 25   Factitious disorder

Relatively little is known about this man but it is thought that he turns up at emergency departments in various parts of the country with false stories of illness in order to obtain treatments. He is an intelligent individual, apparently in his mid-40s, who probably uses different aliases, so it is uncertain whether he is responsible for the very many appearances attributed to him.

For certain periods he specialises in very vivid physical complaints and is known to have had a variety of operations, mainly abdominal. He usually decamps from hospital before he is faced with his lies. He appears to be extraordinarily persuasive and often receives injections of narcotics because he can feign severe pain and distress.

At other times (perhaps while waiting for his latest surgical scar to heal) he appears elsewhere with variations on a story that he has a chronic psychiatric illness. The description he gives is of a florid delusional illness and he says that he receives a depot injection of a neuroleptic to counteract this. He tells staff that he is hitchhiking from one part of the country to another to reach his home, that this is taking much longer than he expected, and that he is beginning to re-experience his abnormal thoughts and hallucinations because his medication is overdue. Because he can quote the exact nature of the depot medication, its dose and the frequency of administration, he is often believed and given the injection. He then says that he is on benztropine and needs a supply to counteract Parkinsonian side effects. He will repeat this performance at fairly short intervals in the different emergency departments of that town before moving on to another location.

From what little that can be put together about this man, he probably does not have a psychotic illness but is willing to have the injections in order to obtain a supply of benztropine, to which he may well be addicted. His elusiveness has prevented adequate tracking and preventive intervention up until now.

Asperger's disorder

Case No. 26   Asperger's disorder

A man aged 23 was remanded to a forensic psychiatric unit for assessment after having been charged with several counts of fraud. At interview he initially created a strange impression. He had a severe left-sided strabismus, his body movements were unco-ordinated and clumsy, he talked in a loud, uninflected voice, and his manner was inappropriately condescending. He readily admitted to the charges against him but said that they were invalid because he was a special person who could use other people's money to carry on his own work as a computer specialist. Otherwise he was not very co-operative in providing a history. A tentative diagnosis of schizophrenia or delusional disorder had been made by the first psychiatrist to see him following the charges.

Eventually, it was learned from members of his family that the patient had always been difficult and eccentric. His birth had been very prolonged and he was difficult to resuscitate. As a small child he was physically unco-ordinated, poor in verbal and communicative skills and socially isolated. Despite ocular surgery he continued to have a strabismus and his vision was extremely myopic. He had required special education and at first was thought to be educationally subnormal. However, it was noted almost accidentally that he had good mathematical skills and these were encouraged. He had progressed to computers and was extremely competent with them, although with an exaggerated view of his abilities.

After finishing school he obtained several computer-related jobs. Provided he was left on his own he could cope with these but as soon as other people were involved he became withdrawn and unco-operative and the jobs were inevitably terminated. Unfortunately, an older individual, a man known to have criminal connections, began to cultivate him and got him to carry out computer projects on his behalf. With his extraordinary naîvete the patient had no idea he was involved in any illegal activities and seemed to have limited understanding of the nature of the accusations against him.

A period of observation revealed no psychotic disorder to be present. He was not deluded although he had inflated ideas about his skills, and his 'grandiosity' was, in fact, his habitual disinhibited behaviour allied with lack of insight. It was agreed by those who observed him in the forensic unit that he should be diagnosed as suffering from Asperger's syndrome.

Eating disorders

Anorexia nervosa may, at times, be associated with extraordinary ideas by the individual about her body shape. These fixations are not usually delusional but on occasion may be (Plantey, 1977; Hudson, Pope and Jonas, 1984; Garfinkel, Kennedy and Caplan, 1995). When this occurs the focus of treatment has to change and the first priority is to deal with the psychosis, whatever specific form it may assume. Interestingly, and quite apart from the presence of psychosis, there is a small literature which appears to show that pimozide in addition to behaviour therapy, or as an alternative to the latter, may bring about significant weight gain in typical cases of anorexia nervosa (Vandereycken and Pierloot, 1982; Weizman and colleagues, 1985).

Case No. 27   Delusional disorder presenting as anorexia nervosa

A 22-year-old female has been anorexic since the age of 14 and has had numerous courses of treatment, including several periods as an inpatient. She has always resisted help and has been regarded throughout as an especially difficult therapeutic problem. In the family background there is a strong history of psychoactive substance abuse and her father is a treated alcoholic.

The patient has always been ultra-preoccupied by body size and shape, and her ideal is to be permanently cachectic. At the age of 20 she was noted to be becoming more withdrawn and her conversation, always laconic, became almost nonexistent. She began to neglect her toilet, refuse help and ignore her already-minute diet. She had to be admitted to a general hospital medical unit to deal with life-threatening starvation. There she refused oral nutrition or medications and had to be treated via intravenous infusions.

On one occasion she was visited by a young female consultation–liaison psychiatrist who sat with her quietly for a considerable time and suddenly the patient began to talk. It emerged that she had a florid, highly involved and quasi-logical delusional system, involving grandiose religious beliefs and a conviction that she was a 'second Messiah who must assume perfect form and then die to redeem the people'. This apotheosis was to be achieved before the year 2000.

She would not talk about this to anyone else, but spoke freely to the female psychiatrist on several occasions, developing her theme with ever-greater elaboration and considerable clarity. She had no insight and pooh-poohed any idea that she was psychologically ill. Apart from her delusional system there was no generalised thought disorder or evidence of wide-ranging delusions. A complex situation ensued with much disagreement about her capacity to accept or reject treatment, but finally and with legal assistance it was decided she was not capable of understanding her illness or the treatment she required for it. Because her anorexia threatened her life and because of wholehearted parental support, treatment with moderate dosages of a neuroleptic was started.

The effect is not dramatic but the patient has become less preoccupied and withdrawn. She has gradually been encouraged to take a limited, but more normal, diet and her weight has moderately increased. She remains mostly at home, will not take part in the eating disorders clinic she used to attend regularly, and accepts her anti-psychotic medication from her family physician. She does not attend church but reads a great deal of religious literature. She never makes reference to her delusional beliefs to her parents or physicians.

Pathological bereavement

Case No. 28   Pathological bereavement

A man of 63 had always been excessively quiet and shy. Rather late in life he married a lady who was much more outgoing and who encouraged him to join her in a number of social activities. He enjoyed these but never made friends and totally depended on her both at home and elsewhere. He gave up his work at the age of 60 with a sense of relief because he always dreaded the social contacts there.

His wife died suddenly of a heart attack about a year after his retirement. He was devastated and thereafter spent most of his time at home, only going out when he had to in order to purchase minimal amounts of food. His relatives eventually became concerned at his severe loss of weight and air of misery, and took him to his family physician. The latter gave him antidepressants for a time but when the patient told him he wished he were dead he arranged for admission to the local psychiatric unit.

There he was found to be a malnourished man who was very withdrawn and sad-looking, yet who, on occasion, would smile in a rather secretive way when asked about his thoughts and feelings. It took a considerable time to obtain his confidence and then he began to talk quite freely, but in a repetitive way and always about his adored wife. He said that nothing else mattered to him but her, that he had built a shrine to her in their bedroom, and every day he spent hours there conversing with her. She often appeared to him as a real-looking, three-dimensional vision, told him that she was in Heaven and said that he was to join her when she gave the signal. She told him that he was to save his pills so that he could kill himself when she said so, and that she could guarantee that this would not be a sin. He said it was only a matter of time until he obeyed her and he had no interest in treatment or in any kind of life without her.

After considerable observation and after reviewing the possibility
that he might be severely depressed, schizophrenic, suffering from a
delusional disorder or an early dementia, all of these possibilities were
finally rejected and it was decided that this was an abnormal grief
reaction in a man with a lifelong schizoid personality who had been
grossly overdependent on his late wife. As a precaution, and with his
agreement, he was given a very adequate trial of another antidepressant but with absolutely no benefit. He was completely unable to enter
into any psychotherapeutic process and an attempt to provide cognitive therapy failed because he had no wish to comply. Finally he was
discharged. Two years later he was still alive and apparently un-
changed, but was refusing any outside help whatsoever.

Conclusion

In psychiatry, nothing substitutes adequately for the combination of a
thorough history (including collateral history), mental and physical examination, and adequate observation over a period of time. On first presentation a psychiatric illness may be almost immediately recognisable but in a
considerable proportion of cases we need time to clarify the diagnosis and
an over-hasty attempt to reach closure may be quite disastrous for some
patients. In the context of this book it is essential that the point be made
that delusional disorder is quite readily mimicked by a variety of other
illnesses.

No doubt the professional reader can supply his or her experience of
other psychiatric illnesses which may easily be mistaken for delusional
disorder. A well-informed clinician with good knowledge of the current
diagnostic canon will be aware of such situations and will make the
minimum of errors in differentiating delusional disorder from its imitators.

References

Diagnostic and Statistical Manual of Mental Disorders, 4th edn (DSMIV) (1994).
 Washington, DC: American Psychiatric Association.
Dorfman, A., Shields, G. and Delisi, L.E. (1993). DSMIIIR personality disorders
 in parents of schizophrenic patients. *Am. J. Med. Genet. (Neuropsychiatric
 Genetics)* **48**: 60–62.
Fulton, M. and Winokur, G. (1993). A comparative study of paranoid and
 schizoid personality disorders. *Am. J. Psychiat.* **150**: 1363–1367.
Garfinkel, P.E., Kennedy, S.H. and Kaplan, A.S. (1995).Views on classification

and diagnosis of eating disorders. *Can. J. Psychiat.* **40**: 445–456.

Hudson, J.I., Pope, H.G. and Jonas, J.M. (1984). Psychosis in anorexia nervosa and bulimia. *Br. J. Psychiat.* **145**: 420–423.

International Statistical Classification of Diseases, 10th edn (ICD10) (1992–3). Geneva: World Health Organization.

Kendler, K.S. and Gruenberg, A.M. (1982). Genetic relationship between paranoid personality disorder and the 'schizophrenic spectrum' disorders. *Am. J. Psychiat.* **139**: 1185–1186.

Kendler, K.S., Masterson, C.C., Ungaro, R. and Davis, K.L. (1984). A family history study of schizophrenia-related personality disorders. *Am. J. Psychiat.* **141**: 424–427.

Lloyd, G.G. (1986). Psychiatric syndromes with a somatic presentation. *J. Psychosom. Res.* **30**: 113–120.

McElroy, S.L., Phillips, K.A., Keck, P.E., Hudson, J.I. and Pope, H.G. (1993). Body dysmorphic disorder: does it have a psychotic subtype? *J. Clin. Psychiat.* **54**: 389–395.

Munro, A. (1982). *Delusional Hypochondriasis*. Clarke Institute of Psychiatry Monograph No. 5. Toronto: Clarke Institute of Psychiatry.

Phillips. K.A. and McElroy, S.L. (1993). Insight, overvalued ideation, and delusional thinking in body dysmorphic disorder: theoretical and treatment implications. *J. Nerv. Ment. Dis.* **181**: 699–702.

Phillips, K.A., McElroy, S.L., Keck, P.E., Pope, H.G. and Hudson, J.I. (1993). Body dysmorphic disorder: 30 cases of imagined ugliness. *Am. J. Psychiat.* **150**: 302–308.

Plantey, F. (1977). Pimozide in treatment of anorexia nervosa. *Lancet*, **1**: 1105 (letter).

Rosen, J.C. (1995). The nature of body dysmorphic disorder and treatment with cognitive behavior therapy. *Cogn. Behav. Pract.* **2**: 143–166.

Vandereycken, W. and Pierloot, R. (1982). Pimozide combined with behaviour therapy in the short-term treatment of anorexia nervosa. *Acta Psychiat. Scand.* **66**: 445–450.

Weizman, A., Tyano, S., Wüsenbeek, H. and Ben David, M. (1985). Behavior therapy, pimozide treatment and prolactin secretion in anorexia nervosa. *Psychother. Psychosom.* **43**: 136–140.

Winokur, G. (1985). Familial psychopathology in delusional disorder. *Comp. Psychiat.* **26**: 241–248.

Part V
Treatment of delusional disorder and overall conclusions

It takes as much time and trouble to pull down a falsehood as to build up a truth.
Peter Mere Latham (1789–1875)

When paranoia and the other paranoid spectrum disorders were widely-accepted diagnostic entities, there was no effective treatment for any psychiatric illness. There were many 'therapies' but, unless the illness was self-limiting, few if any therapeutic successes.

While paranoia was in abeyance for many years as a recognized illness, useful treatments began to appear in psychiatry and many illnesses which were previously regarded as hopeless are now readily treatable. Unhappily, when DSMIIIRs description of delusional disorder revived our awareness of paranoia, it somehow failed to dispel the nihilistic view of treatment which had been justified 50 years before.

Nowadays, delusional disorder is treatable, often highly treatable, but it has to be recognized that the patient has to be persuaded to comply with treatment, and the treatment must be appropriate. The burden of Chapter 13 is to describe the treatment of this illness in modern, realistic but optimistic terms. Admittedly there is little scientific content as yet, but there is more consensus on methodology than many professionals realise. Delusional disorder is not a pleasant illness and it behoves the clinician to know enough about it to give the patient his or her best chance of effective therapy.

The brain is beginning to deliver its secrets to modern technologies and the delusional disorders – all of them – may well benefit from this process. We desperately need a scientific underpinning to the subject which will be worthy of the twenty-first century. The concluding chapter provides some thoughts on this aspect.

13

The treatment of delusional disorder

In 1975, Riding and Munro reported on the successful treatment of five cases of monodelusional hypochondriacal psychosis (MHP) (now more often referred to as delusional disorder, somatic subtype), and in 1982 the present author followed this up with a report of a further 45 cases. Since then there has been an increasing number of communications regarding the successful treatment of the different subtypes of delusional disorder, unfortunately most of them on an anecdotal basis, but overall adding up to a refutation of the belief that delusional disorder is irremediable. Virtually all of these reports refer to psychopharmacological treatment.

Treatment of delusions in general

To be accurate, we rarely attempt to treat a delusion by itself but rather the illness of which it is a part, although there is a respectable psychological literature showing that delusions *per se*, as well as hallucinations, can be considerably modified by, for example, cognitive–behavioural therapy (Chadwick and Birchwood, 1994; Garety and Hemsley, 1994; Kingdon, Turkington and John, 1994). Psychotic disorders characterized by delusions are usually treated by neuroleptic medications or, in some cases, with electroconvulsive therapy and careful diagnosis is required to determine which treatments are most appropriate. We usually expect the delusions to improve as the underlying illness resolves although, as noted in Chapter 7 on paraphrenia, they can often be much more persistent than we realise.

In Chapter 2 we discussed illnesses associated with delusions. In addition to delusional disorder itself, the following delusional conditions were noted as most important in differential diagnosis:

Paraphrenia
Paranoid schizophrenia
Other schizophrenias
Organic mental disorders, including delirium, dementia or those due to a
  general medical condition
Psychoactive substance-related organic mental disorders
Mood disorders with delusions
Psychotic disorders not otherwise specified
Delusional misidentification syndromes
Shared psychotic disorder (induced delusional disorder or *folie à deux*)
Schizoaffective disorder

In the above list, paraphrenia, paranoid schizophrenia and other schizophrenias, psychotic disorders not otherwise specified, and schizoaffective
disorder, will usually be treated primarily with neuroleptics, conventional
or atypical. In addition, schizoaffective disorder may warrant simultaneous treatment with neuroleptics, antidepressant drugs, mood-stabilisers
or even electroconvulsive therapy.

Organic mental disorders may also require neuroleptic treatment: in
delirium, haloperidol is often effective in controlling psychotic thinking
and behaviour, and it and other neuroleptics may be successful in reducing
the intensity of delusions in dementing disorders and in mental disorders
secondary to a general medical condition. Anticonvulsants may also play a
part in such situations.

Mood disorders with delusions can be treated with a combination of
antidepressant and neuroleptic drugs or with electroconvulsive therapy. In
the delusional misidentification syndromes, neuroleptics are sometimes
useful but Spier (1992) suggests that anticonvulsants should be considered
as adjunctive or even primary medications in such cases.

In shared psychotic disorder, treatment is by successfully controlling the
delusions in the primary patient with neuroleptic medication or by separating the primary and secondary individuals (see Chapter 10). In the less
usual cases of *folie simultanée*, the two individuals need to be treated with
antipsychotic drugs.

Opler, Klahr and Ramirez (1995) remind us that the rate of symptom
response to treatment in any psychiatric disorder may not be uniform.
Hallucinations often begin to improve fairly rapidly but, as noted, delusions frequently persist for many months and, in a proportion of cases,
never remit fully. (The present author's colleagues, Drs Ravindran and
Yatham have certainly found this to be very true of paraphrenia – see

Chapter 7.) This means that patients leaving hospital after apparently successful antipsychotic treatment may still be actively deluded, and this is probably an important factor in subsequent noncompliance with treatment. Opler, Klahr and Ramirez (1995) suggest, in fact, that delusions may be linked to underlying pathologies which are different from those provoking other psychotic symptoms, and this opinion may have some validity.

Treatment of paranoia/delusional disorder

The present author (Munro, 1982) has presented evidence that what we now call delusional disorder of the somatic subtype is a highly treatable disorder. Among the described cases, those which failed to improve were, in some instances, very likely to be noncompliant with medication and it has since emerged that noncompliance with psychiatric treatment is a common feature of delusional disorder in general. Getting the patient to see a psychiatrist and getting him or her to accept psychotropic medication are extremely difficult processes, and even when patients do agree to take drugs, a proportion actually fail to follow through.

In the past two decades, there have been many reports, internationally, describing the treatment of the somatic subtype of delusional disorder with psychotropic drugs. As previously mentioned, Riding and Munro (1975) described the successful treatment of five cases of this condition, using the diphenylbutylpiperidine drug, pimozide and a later report (Munro, 1982) expanded on the employment of pimozide. Since then, this has proved to be the most common drug of first choice for this subtype (Munro and Mok, 1995).

More recently, reports on the treatment of jealousy, erotomanic and persecutory subtypes have appeared (see Chapters 4–6). It is a great pity that much of the literature here also remains anecdotal, and results are usually based on single case outcomes or on very small series, but outcome trend is similar to that of cases with somatic delusions.

One reason for the lack of scientific evidence on the treatment of delusional disorder is the notorious reluctance of delusional disorder patients to engage in psychotropic drug trials. Their inherent suspiciousness and specific rejection of psychiatrists make actual treatment difficult enough, never mind a medication study. This writer has learned this the hard way, in failing to get a simple comparison between pimozide and chlorpromazine under way due to lack of patient co-operation. However, three small systematic trials seem to have confirmed pimozide's particular usefulness in the somatic subtype (Hamann and Avnstorp, 1982; Lindskov and Baadsgaard, 1985; Ungvári and Vladár, 1986). Interestingly, dermatologists are enthusiastically employing pimozide to treat delusions of skin infestation since Lyell (1983) described its efficacy (Reilly and Batchelor, 1986; Koo and Strauss, 1987; Van Moffaert, 1992).

When a colleague and the present writer set out to review the world literature on the treatment of delusional disorder (Munro and Mok, 1995), approximately 1000 articles were sifted in detail, dating from 1961 but with the great majority dating from 1980 onwards. Sadly, it was found that case descriptions were often extremely vague or nonexistent and, since only patients whose illness was recognisable according to DSMIV were accepted, many cases had to be rejected. In the article, the writings from which results had been extracted were carefully listed, as well as those whose contents were unsuitable for analysis, to provide other workers with an opportunity to confirm or refute the authors' assertions. Because of the poor quality of much of the information obtained it was only possible to describe rather broad categories of response to treatment, i.e., 'recovery', 'partial recovery', 'no improvement' and, where applicable, 'noncompliance'. The results of pimozide were compared with those of a mixed group of other neuroleptics, numbers being too small to individualise these other drugs' effects.

The authors were able to extract details of 257 cases which satisfied the DSMIV criteria for delusional disorder but, of these, adequate treatment details were obtainable in only 209 individuals, 50 of whom had previously been reported by the present author (Munro, 1982). It was noted that, prior to 1980, a variety of neuroleptics was employed in treatment but that, since 1980, pimozide was the most common single drug of choice. In some cases two or more drugs had been employed but authors usually failed to provide details of the time sequence.

From a meta-analysis it was first of all possible to determine that the broad characteristics of the patients were compatible with the general description of individuals with delusional disorder (Munro and Chmara, 1982; DSMIV, 1994). For example, females outnumbered males in a proportion of 3:2, on average patients were middle-aged (although the age distribution was from adolescence to extreme old age), and the mean age of the females was greater than that of the males at the time of case identification. Celibacy was common, especially in males, and widowhood was notably high in the women. A positive family history of psychiatric disorder was found in 18.7 per cent of patients but this was regarded as a gross underestimate because of incomplete reporting. A combination of organic brain disorder and/or alcohol or substance abuse was relatively more common among males than among females.

In the literature reviewed, delusional disorder of the somatic subtype is at present the one most frequently recorded, but that is an artefact due to readier recognition of this condition, and probably in no way realistically reflects the relative frequency of the various subtypes. The other traditional themes such as jealousy, erotomania and persecution are beginning to appear increasingly and reflect a similar pattern of treatment outcome. Follow-up information was enormously variable in quality and with a huge time range: from several days to – in one case – 36 years.

Treatment outcome in 209 delusional disorder cases (Munro and Mok, 1995)

Recovery was defined as 'return to full function with total or near-total remission of symptoms'. Partial recovery was 'partial remission of symptoms, significant reduction of anguish and reasonable social adjustment'. No improvement was 'little or no response, continued distress and poor social adjustment'. Noncompliance was recorded when an author clearly indicated its occurrence.

When treatment with all medications combined was studied, it was found that recovery occurred in 110 (52.6 per cent), partial recovery in 59 (28.2 per cent) and no improvement had been noted in 40 (19.2 per cent). When the recovery and partial recovery results were combined, a total of 80.8 per cent of the patients were included. The present author (Munro, 1982) had previously found that 41 of his 50 delusional disorder cases showed 'excellent' or 'fair' outcome, an almost identical overall result.

Mok and this writer considered the effects of pimozide separately from those of all other neuroleptics combined, and an interesting and significant difference emerged between pimozide and these other neuroleptics. Of 143 individuals treated with pimozide, 98 (68.5 per cent) were judged to have recovered fully and 32 (22.4 per cent) partially, making a total of 90.9 per cent with a greater or lesser degree of improvement. (In the author's own series noted above, all treated with pimozide, the figures were 32 (64 per cent) and 9 (18 per cent), respectively – again remarkably similar.) The 53 patients treated with one of several other neuroleptics showed 12 (22.6 per cent) with full recovery and 24 (45.3 per cent) with partial recovery, a total of 67.9 per cent overall. Comparison indicated that outcome with pimozide was significantly better than that with the other drugs (p 0.001).

Among the recorded instances of noncompliance, 13 in all, none showed recovery, 3 (23.1 per cent) showed partial recovery and 10 (76.9 per cent) no improvement.

The dose of pimozide ranged from 2 mg per day to 40 mg per day, the usual range being 2–16 mg daily. Only two patients received 20 mg or more per day. The other neuroleptics which could be identified were thioridazine, haloperidol, trifluoperazine, loxapine, fluphenazine, sulpiride, chlorprothixene and flupenthixol. In a number of reports it was only possible to say that the neuroleptics were 'unspecified'. Details in the literature were often very sketchy and it was frequently unclear whether adequate dosages of these drugs were always being prescribed.

Another comparison was between the treatment of cases of the somatic subtype on the one hand, and of the persecutory, erotomanic and jealousy subtypes combined, on the other. This was done because, comparatively speaking, the reports on the somatic subtype are better substantiated than are those of the remaining subtypes. No significant difference emerged but the numbers in the second category are small (which is why they were combined), so this result should be interpreted cautiously. Nevertheless, it does seem likely that all the varieties of delusional disorder respond to adequate treatment in approximately the same way.

Incidentally, it seems likely that noncompliance is not always recognized or recorded, and that some cases of 'no improvement' or 'partial recovery' are actually due to lack of co-operation in taking medication. If so, the improvement figures which were found are likely to err on the conservative side.

Practical aspects of treatment

Because many delusional disorder patients are very reluctant to trust a psychiatrist or to accept neuroleptic treatment, ideally it would be best if the assessment and treatment could be carried out by, for example, the family physician, but that presumes some degree of familiarity with the condition and its management on the part of the latter.

Whoever treats these patients needs great patience and it is not uncommon to have to spend more than one session gaining their confidence and finally persuading them to give medication a trial. In their arguments – usually vehement and often very well presented – all kinds of sophistry are employed to avoid accepting a neuroleptic, but calm persistence does finally pay off in a reasonable proportion of cases.

It is the author's unvarying custom to start with a very low dose of neuroleptic, for example, usually prescribing pimozide as the drug of first choice and starting with 1 or 2 mg daily. Thereafter, the dose is raised gradually and cautiously and in most cases need go no higher than 4 to 6 mg per day. That way, there is no sudden onset of side effects, an event guaranteed to induce immediate noncompliance. The patient should be seen at least once a week during this early stage and, if he or she is being compliant and the medication is successful, it is not unusual to see minor improvements within a few days, such as reduced agitation, a slight improvement in morale, better sleep or somewhat reduced preoccupation with the delusion, whether it be hypochondriacal, persecutory, erotomanic, or other. On average, it takes about two weeks of continuous, adequate treatment to produce significant amelioration of the delusion, but in some patients it may be six weeks or longer.

Quite often the patient feels sufficiently improved early on in treatment that he or she decides to stop the medication. Inevitably the delusion and the accompanying agitation and preoccupation start to reappear and it is then that the treating physician has the best opportunity to obtain ongoing co-operation. Even when the patient is still adamant that his beliefs are real, the experience of improvement followed by incipient relapse seems to make a deep impression and if the patient now trusts the physician he or she will often become extremely compliant. In successful cases the complete turnaround from rejection to trust is both remarkable and heartily gratifying.

One striking observation is that, when delusional disorder patients make a good recovery, this is often relatively rapid and notably complete. This is true even when the delusion has been present for a very long time. One has been impressed on many occasions that, following recovery, the individual is often strikingly well functioning, with little evidence of the personality disorder that is supposed to be a premorbid feature of so many cases of delusional disorder, and requiring little psychotherapeutic or other help to resume a more normal everyday life. This has led the writer to speculate that perhaps what is interpreted as antecedent personality disorder (even by patients themselves) may be a very prolonged prodromal phase of the delusional illness itself (see Chapter 2).

Maintenance of treatment

We are dealing with a potentially life-long illness and it would therefore not be surprising to find that treatment might need to be continued indefinitely. We have virtually no objective information on this. The writer has maintained contact with several patients for up to four years, and one for ten years. About one-third of these longer follow-up patients have been successfully weaned from their treatment, but it is interesting that they themselves then keep a look-out for recurrence of symptoms and, in a small number of cases, it has been noted that tension-inducing situations will sometimes provoke a minor recurrence. For example, a former infestation delusion patient will begin to notice a skin itch, and a patient who had had persecutory delusions will start to feel suspicious about other people again. (A man with jealousy delusions which responded well to treatment would telephone the writer from time to time saying, 'Doctor, I'm beginning to have funny thoughts about my wife again. Should I put the dose back up?') If this minor recurrence happens repeatedly, a few patients will ask to be reinstated on regular doses of neuroleptic.

The patient who has been followed for ten years had a persecutory subtype with somewhat grandiose overtones. Several times in these ten years she has taken herself off the neuroleptic and invariably, after a few weeks, her symptoms insidiously begin to reappear and she and her husband agree that she has to resume her medication. Unfortunately we have no predictive criteria at present to tell us which patients should be able to terminate treatment safely in the course of time.

There is a dissociation between acquired insight as to the desirability of continuing treatment and in-depth insight into the illness itself. Many patients never accept fully the psychotic nature of their experience, but so long as they agree to take treatment, it seems unimportant, and probably unkind, to face them with the fact that they were delusional before the medication took effect.

Non-drug treatment of delusional disorder

There is evidence that cognitive–behavioural therapy may be capable of modifying delusions (see p.32), but none which suggests that psychological approaches are effective in treating actual delusional disorder. At present, much psychological skill and diplomacy is essential in engaging the patient but thereafter, treatment is exclusively psychopharmacological until the delusion is largely resolved. Thereafter, psychological help may be valuable in guiding some patients who require it back to a productive lifestyle, and that may be cognitive–behavioural or psychodynamic according to the requirement (Kingdon, Turkington and John, 1994; Fear, Sharp and Healy, 1996). There is a general consensus that psychotherapy of an exploratory, uncovering type is not appropriate in delusional disorder.

Post-psychotic depression

In the author's personal series, 6 out of 50 treated patients experienced marked depressive symptoms while receiving a neuroleptic. Various explanations for this are possible. For example, it could be seen as a drug side effect or could be interpreted more psychologically. These individuals have been totally committed to their delusional belief, sometimes for many years, and the sudden remission of their symptoms seems to catch them totally unprepared. In some cases a marked lability of mood, and in others a fixed depression, appears and, in the midst of this, it may be that some patients are depressed because they find it difficult to cope with the painful revelation that, if their improvement is due to an antipsychotic drug, they must have been 'insane'.

On the whole it seems likely that this type of post-psychotic depression is actually a neurochemical phenomenon in most instances, and it is not restricted to the recovery phase of delusional disorder. DSMIV has a tentative category of post-schizophrenic depression, not yet made official, and this is a well-known phenomenon to practising clinicians. Since delusional disorder was not amenable to treatment until lately, depression could never be observed in its recovery. Now it has been, and DSMIV and ICD10 would be well advised to have a recognized category, but to name it post-psychotic, rather than just post-schizophrenic, depressive disorder.

In this writer's early experience of it, it was assumed to be a drug side effect and it seemed logical to stop the neuroleptic. Invariably the depression lifted but the original delusions recurred. The proper approach is to continue with the minimum effective dose of the neuroleptic and to add a therapeutic dose of an antidepressant drug. After an appropriate time has elapsed, the latter can usually be weaned off.

It is very important to stress that post-psychotic depression is not uncommon and is potentially dangerous since some patients begin to exhibit suicidal thinking. Psychiatrists must therefore keep a close watch for its appearance in the recovering schizophrenic or delusional disorder patient.

Choice of medication in the treatment of delusional disorder

The present author's interest in delusional disorder originally arose because of the serendipitous response of a small number of patients with the somatic subtype to the administration of pimozide. Since the condition was reputedly untreatable and since the results were so dramatically good, one was encouraged to go on seeking similar cases and treating them with the same medication. Also, many of the patients who were seen and treated reported having previously received benzodiazepines, antidepressants or other neuroleptics for the treatment of their disorder, but with no success. When pimozide worked – and it so often did – it seemed that it had therapeutic advantages over these other drugs. As noted, other people have used it and have reported good success (Tueth and Cheong, 1993; Opler, Klahr and Ramirez, 1995).

However, there is very little scientific evidence to support pimozide or any other specific medication's particular effectiveness in delusional disorder. As explained, this is due to a combination of the difficulty in obtaining extended case-series, and the inherent unwillingness of delusional disorder patients to enter scientific drug trials. The three small studies on record (see p.230) do appear to reflect that pimozide is highly effective and, again, it has to be remembered that this effectiveness is occurring in an illness which is both extremely chronic and reputedly untreatable.

When Mok and the author (Munro and Mok, 1995) reported on our review findings, we were well aware of the numerous methodological faults in the literature we studied. There is no question that research on delusional disorder in general needs to be radically improved as far as scientific scrupulousness is concerned. Another concern was that, because of the present author's published work on the use of primozide in delusional disorder, this drug has nowadays definitely become the first choice for treatment by psychiatrists (and dermatologists – see p.230). Therefore, reports about other neuroleptics tend to be in older articles and this makes comparison between them and pimozide more uncertain.

One must be prepared to agree that the use of pimozide in delusional disorder is being encouraged by a number of enthusiasts, the present writer included. There is also concern that, in the review by Mok and Munro, we are comparing one drug (pimozide) with a collection of other drugs: this may be unfair since an unfavourable group effect among the latter may conceal the superior action of a small number of others. Nevertheless, it does appear that the results of treatment with pimozide exhibit a higher preponderance of good outcomes and this suggests, though it certainly does not prove, that pimozide is probably the logical first-line approach for delusional disorder at this time. It should be noted that, as already pointed out, whatever the neuroleptic used, it will require long-term, and possibly permanent, administration and, at least to begin with, close supervision.

An interesting suggestion has recently been made by a psychiatric colleague, Dr Lili Kopala, about the apparent success of pimozide in delusional disorder. Dr Kopala has published authoritative research results on the successful use of low-dose neuroleptics in previously untreated schizophrenic patients (Kopala and colleagues, 1996; Kopala, Good and Honer, 1997). This writer has always advocated the use of low-dose pimozide in delusional disorder, partly to reduce side effects and enhance compliance, and partly because experience has shown that relatively low doses (rarely more than 6 mg per day of this powerful drug) are effective. Dr Kopala has hypothesised that the success of pimozide might actually be due to this low-dose approach, with larger doses masking any positive effect. And, of course, it is not unlikely that other neuroleptics would have been given in relatively heroic dosages, possibly appropriate to schizophrenia but certainly not to delusional disorder. This is a viewpoint which may well merit further consideration and experimentation.

Because of the delusional disorder patient's excessive wariness and suspicion, conventional double-blind drug trials may be all but impossible. If, on the other hand, co-operation can be gained from single individuals, perhaps a within-patient comparison of the effect of different drugs may be feasible: that is, the $N = 1$ approach (Klieser and Wolfrum, 1985). One great advantage of delusional disorder patients as experimental subjects, if they can be persuaded to co-operate, is that they are usually not taking a neuroleptic drug at the time of first presentation, so they represent that commodity which is so rare nowadays, a population of drug-naïve individuals.

If no other conclusion can be reached from the literature to date, the one which must be emphasized again and again is that delusional disorder, properly diagnosed and adequately treated, has an optimistic outlook. Whatever the neuroleptic employed, the overall rate of response, total or partial, is approximately 80 per cent, an outcome that compares well with any other in psychiatry. It is clearly desirable to identify and, if possible, treat cases.

What is sad is that some psychiatrists, presumably due to unfamiliarity, still do not really recognize delusional disorder. Also, despite warnings that relatively low doses of neuroleptic seem to be most appropriate in this illness, we still find reports of patients being treated with high levels of medication which must be detrimental to their general health and probably counterproductive in the attempt to suppress their symptoms.

No clinician should be wedded unthinkingly to some particular form of treatment, but the most persuasive evidence at present, such as it is, is that pimozide is the best documented and most cost effective intervention in delusional disorder. If, at any time, another drug proves to be superior to pimozide then let us move to its use immediately. In the meantime, if only for the wretched patients' sake, one must make the strongest of pleas that the illness be diagnosed accurately and that it be treated with 'state of the art' efficiency.

Pimozide – mechanisms, side effects and uses

Quite apart from its putative usefulness in delusional disorder, pimozide is an interesting and versatile drug. First discovered by Janssen in the 1960s (Janssen and colleagues, 1968) it was developed as a conventional anti-psychotic medication. It remains one of the purest antidopaminergic drugs in our armamentarium, and much of the blocking of dopamine effects is post-synaptic (Walter and Roth, 1976; Chouinard and Annable, 1982). It has a low affinity for alpha-receptors, so there is a relative lack of noradrenergic blockade (Opler and Feinberg, 1991) and a low incidence of sedation or orthostatic hypotension (Peroutka and colleagues, 1977). In general, its side effects are relatively benign (Shapiro, Shapiro and Eisenkraft, 1983). Usually, it can be given in a single dose each day.

However, pimozide has a significant calcium channel antagonist action (Qar, Galizzi and Fossett, 1987), and this has been blamed for the phenomenon of prolongation of the QT interval in the electrocardiogram (ECG) of about 10 per cent of patients treated with pimozide (Fulop and colleagues, 1986). In the United States, the Federal Drug Agency has recommended that patients being treated with pimozide have a pretreatment ECG and periodic follow-up ECGs, especially when the dose is being increased, but Tueth and Cheong (1993) note that on normal dosage schedules the risk of cardiac decompensation is very slight.

Another aspect of the drug is its interaction with opiate receptors (Creese, Feinberg and Snyder, 1976), and this has been linked to the mildly euphoriant effect that pimozide has in some individuals (Hoehe, Duka and Doeniche, 1988).

Possibly because of its relative lack of presynaptic antidopaminergic activity, pimozide does not usually prove effective in the treatment of acutely agitated schizophrenic patients: this is interesting, since one of its early benefits in agitated delusional disorder is a calming effect. Side effects can include extrapyramidal symptoms but in the low doses used in delusional disorder, pimozide is usually much more benign in this respect than other conventional neuroleptics and it has also been used successfully, with few deleterious effects, in the longer-term treatment of negative symptom schizophrenics (Feinberg and colleagues, 1988). Tueth and Cheong (1993) actually propose that pimozide should be given a trial in chronic negative-symptom schizophrenic patients before giving a drug like clozapine, which has, of course, potentially devastating side effects in a small subgroup of treated patients (McKenna and Bailey, 1993).

At the present time, pimozide is widely used as a treatment for Gilles de la Tourette syndrome (Regeur, Pakkenberg and Pakkenberg, 1986; Shapiro, Shapiro and Fulop, 1987), for delusional disorder (Opler, Klahr and Ramirez, 1995), for the treatment of negative-symptom schizophrenia (Tueth and Cheong, 1993), for post herpetic neuralgia (Duke, 1983), and for trigeminal neuralgia (Lechin and colleagues, 1989). An additional and intriguing use is in the treatment of melanomatous metastases which are apparently dopamine-driven in some cases (Neifeld and colleagues, 1983).

As already described, there are reports of the effectiveness of pimozide in virtually all of the subtypes of delusional disorder (see Chapters 5–8). One of the most widely accepted uses of the drug is in the treatment of delusions of parasitosis (Reilly and Batchelor, 1986; van Moffaert, 1992; Baker, Cook and Winokur, 1995). With reference to this, Botschev and Müller (1991) suggest that pimozide may be particularly effective because it stimulates the individual's opiate receptors and produces an endorphin-like effect, with euphoria and decreased itchiness and, subsequently, diminution of the delusion. This is an interesting observation and perhaps the itch in the somatic subtype does respond directly to pimozide's action, but this does not explain the apparently equal effectiveness of the drug in delusions of jealousy, erotomania, dysmorphia, etc.

Conclusion

Every psychiatrist familiar with DSMIV and ICD10 should be able to recognize and diagnose delusional disorder. He or she should also be competent to deal with an illness which, as will again be emphasized, is eminently treatable if the patient can be persuaded to comply. Ignore those out-of-date comments which still crop up, that it is untreatable: if the clinician works hard to gain the patient's trust, compliance can be obtained in a considerable proportion of cases. Even if pimozide's use is not strongly supported by good scientific evidence as yet, neither is our treatment in many other areas of psychiatric illness. Pimozide is, at the present time, the most widely used drug, and the most common drug of first choice, in delusional disorder. The recommendation is to employ it until something better comes along, but to use it wisely. It is crucial that it be started at a low dose (1–2 mg daily) and gradually raised, but only if need be. There should be a very good reason for giving more than 6 mg/day in delusional disorder.

Treatment aspects of delusional disorder are in crying need of good, experimentally-based drug trials. With new and atypical neuroleptics appearing in increasing numbers, some of them with far less troublesome side effects than their predecessors, there is a promising field here for comparison of their effectiveness against pimozide and other antipsychotics.

Finally, with regard to treatment, it will be remembered that, in Chapter 9, a strong case was made for aligning the delusional misidentification syndromes (DMSs) with the delusional disorders in a combined diagnostic category. It was mentioned there that a small number of reports found pimozide effective in the treatment of DMS, an interesting parallel with the treatment of delusional disorder. However, where substantial organic brain factors appear to be relevant in an individual case of DMS, an anticonvulsant may be the treatment of choice. Since it has been noted (see Chapter 2) that brain abnormalities may be presumed in some cases of paranoia/delusional disorder, one must wonder whether there are some patients with delusional disorder who could benefit from medications like valproic acid or carbamazepine, either alone or in combination with a neuroleptic.

References

Baker, P.B., Cook, B.L. and Winokur,G. (1995). Delusional infestation: the interface of delusions and hallucinations. *Psychiat. Clin. N. Am.* **18**: 345–361.

Botschev, C. and Muller, N. (1991). Opiate receptor antagonists for delusions of parasitosis. *Biol. Psychiat.* **30**: 530 (letter).

Chadwick, P. and Birchwood, M. (1994). The omnipotence of voices: a cognitive approach to auditory hallucinations. *Br. J. Psychiat.* **164**: 190–201.

Chouinard, G. and Annable, L. (1982). Pimozide in the treatment of newly admitted schizophrenic patients. *Psychopharmacology* **76**: 13–19.

Creese, I., Feinberg, A.P. and Snyder, S.H. (1976). Butyrophenone influence on the opiate receptor. *Eur. J. Pharmacol.* **136**: 231–235.

Diagnostic and statistical manual of mental disorders, 4th edn. (DSMIV) (1994). Washington, DC: American Psychiatric Association.

Duke, E.E. (1983). Clinical experience with pimozide: emphasis on its use in postherpetic neuralgia. *J. Am. Acad. Dermatol.* **8**: 845–850.

Fear, C., Sharp, H. and Healy, D. (1996). Cognitive processes in delusional disorders. *Br. J. Psychiat.* **168**: 61–67.

Feinberg, S.S., Kay, S.R., Elijovich, L.R., Fiszbein, A. and Opler, L.A. (1988). Pimozide treatment of the negative schizophrenic syndrome: an open trial. *J.*

Clin. Psychiat. **49**: 235–238.

Fulop, G., Phillips, R., Shapiro, A.K., Gomes, J.A., Shapiro, E. and Nordlie, J.W. (1986). Electrocardiographic changes during haloperidol and pimozide treatment of Tourette's disorder. *Ann. Neurol.* **20**: 437–438.

Garety, P.A. and Hemsley, D.R. (1994). *Delusions: Investigations into the Psychology of Delusional Reasoning.* Maudsley Monograph No. 36. Oxford: Oxford University Press.

Hamann, K. and Avnstorp, C. (1982). Delusions of infestation treated by pimozide: a double-blind crossover clinical study. *Acta Derm. Venereol. (Stockh.)* **62**: 364–366.

Hoehe, M., Duka, T. and Doeniche, A. (1988). Human studies on the 'mu' opiate receptor against fentanyl: neuroendocrine and behavioral responses. *Psychoneuroendocrinology* **13**: 397–408.

International Statistical Classification of Diseases, 10th rev. (ICD10) (1992–93). Geneva: World Health Organization.

Janssen, P.A.J., Niemegeers, C.J.E., Schellekens, K.H.L. Dresse, A., Lenaerts, F.M., Pinchard, A., Schaper, W.K.A., Van Nueten, J.M. and Verbruggen, F.J. (1968). Pimozide, a chemically novel, highly potent and orally long-acting neuroleptic drug. *Arzneimittelforschung* **18**: 261–287.

Kingdon, D., Turkington, D. and John, C. (1994). Cognitive behaviour therapy of schizophrenia. *Br. J. Psychiat.* **164**: 581–587.

Kleiser, E. and Wolfrum, C. (1985). Comparing the effects of pimozide and placebo in a single case experiment. *Pharmacopsychiatry* **18**: 339–342.

Koo, J.Y.M. and Strauss, G.D. (1987). Psychopharmacologic treatment of psychocutaneous disorders: a practical guide. *Sem. Dermatol.* **6**: 83–93.

Kopala, L.C., Fredrikson, K.P., Good, K.P. and Honer, W.G. (1996). Symptoms in neuroleptic-naïve, first-episode schizophrenia: response to risperidone. *Biol. Psychiat.* **39**: 296–298.

Kopala, L.C., Good, K.P. and Honer, W.G. (1997). Extrapyramidal signs and clinical symptoms in first episode schizophrenia: response to low dose risperidone. *J. Clin Psychopharm.* **17**: 308–313.

Lechin, F., Vanderdijs, B., Lechin, M.E., Amat, J., Lechin, A.E., Cabrera, A. *at al.* (1989). Pimozide therapy for trigeminal neuralgia. *Arch. Neurol.* **46**: 960–963.

Lindskov, R. and Baadsgaard, O. (1985). Delusions of infestation treated with pimozide: a follow-up study. *Acta Derm. Venereol. (Stockh.)* **65**: 267–270.

Lyell, A. (1983). Delusions of parasitosis. *Sem. Dermatol.* **2**: 189–195.

McKenna, P.J. and Bailey, P.E. (1993). The strange story of clozapine. *Br. J. Psychiat.* **162**: 32–37.

Munro, A. (1982). *Delusional Hypochondriasis.* Clarke Institute of Psychiatry Monograph No. 5. Toronto: Clarke Institute of Psychiatry.

Munro, A. and Chmara, J. (1982). Monosymptomatic hypochondriacal psychosis: a diagnostic checklist based on 50 cases of the disorder. *Can. J. Psychiat.* **27**: 374–376.

Munro, A. and Mok, H. (1995). An overview of treatment in paranoia/delusional disorder. *Can. J. Psychiat.* **40**: 616–622.

Neifeld, J.P., Tormey, D.C., Baker, M.A., Meyskens, F.L. and Taub, R.N. (1983). Phase II trial of the dopaminergic inhibitor pimozide in previously treated melanoma patients. *Cancer Treat. Rep.* **67**: 155–157.

Opler, L.A. and Feinberg, S.S. (1991). The role of pimozide in clinical psychiatry: a review. *J. Clin. Psychiat.* **52**: 221–233.

Opler, L.A., Klahr, D.M. and Ramirez, P.M. (1995). Pharmacologic treatment of delusions. *Psychiat. Clin. N. Am.* **18**: 379–391.

Peroutka, S.J., U'Prichard, D.C. and Greenberg, D.A. (1977). Neuroleptic drug interactions with norepinephrine alpha receptor binding sites in rat brain. *Neuropharmacology* **16**: 549–556.

Qar, J., Galizzi, J-P. and Fossett, M. (1987). Receptors for diphenylbutylpiperidine neuroleptic in brain, cardiac and smooth muscle membranes: relationship with receptors for 1,4–dihydropyridines and phenylalkylamines and with Ca2+ channel blockade. *Eur. J. Pharmacol.* **141**: 261–268.

Regeur, L., Pakkenberg, B., Fog, R. and Pakkenberg, H. (1986). Clinical features and long-term treatment with pimozide in 65 patients with Gilles de la Tourette's syndrome. *J. Neurol. Neurosurg. Psychiat.* **49**: 791–795.

Reilly, T.M. and Batchelor, D.H. (1986). The presentation and treatment of delusional parasitosis: a dermatological perspective. *Int. Clin. Psychopharmacol.* **1**: 340–353.

Riding, J. and Munro, A. (1975). Pimozide in the treatment of monosymptomatic hypochondriacal psychosis. *Acta Psychiat. Scand.* **52**: 23–30.

Shapiro, A.K., Shapiro, E. and Eisenkraft, G.J. (1983).Treatment of Gilles de la Tourette syndrome with pimozide. *Am. J. Psychiat.* **140**: 1183–1186.

Shapiro, A.K., Shapiro, E. and Fulop, G. (1987). Pimozide treatment of tic and Tourette disorders. *Pediatrics* **79**: 1032–1039.

Spier, S.A. (1992). Capgras' syndrome and the delusions of misidentification. *Psychiat. Ann.* **22**: 279–285.

Tueth, M.J. and Cheong, J.A. (1993). Clinical uses of pimozide. *Southern Med. J.* **86**: 344–349.

Ungvári, G. and Vladár, K. (1986). Pimozide treatment for delusion of infestation. *Activ. Nerv. Sup. (Prague)* **28**: 103–107.

Van Moffaert, M. (1992). Psychodermatology: an overview. *Psychother. Psychosom.* **58**: 125–136.

Walter, J.R. and Roth, R.H. (1976). Dopaminergic neurons: an in vivo system for measuring drug interactions with presynaptic receptors. *Arch. Pharmacol.* **296**: 5–14.

Warwick, H.M., Clark, D.M., Cobb, A.M. and Salkovskis, P.M. (1996). A controlled trial of cognitive-behavioural treatment of hypochondriasis. *Br. J. Psychiat.* **169**: 189–195.

14
Conclusions

Life is the art of drawing sufficient conclusions from insufficient premises.
Samuel Butler (1835–1902)

The dogmas of the quiet past are inadequate to the stormy present.
Abraham Lincoln (1809–1865)

Introduction

This book has had two main purposes. The first has been to gather together what we know about delusional disorder, to try to put it into some kind of systematic and understandable order, and then dare the reader to improve upon it. The second is to hammer home the point that this is a very real illness which causes a great deal of suffering and to insist that it is an onus on every psychiatrist to be able to diagnose it properly and treat it adequately.

With reference to the two quotations at the beginning of this chapter: much of our past knowledge on delusional disorder is little more than dogma and our current information is still so flimsy that any conclusions we draw from it can only be seen as ephemeral – to be challenged by new data as they appear. It is hoped that potential researchers in the field of delusional disorder will not be discouraged by the backward state of our knowledge and will keep Mary Queen of Scots' motto in mind: 'In my end is my beginning.'

Delusional disorder lay rusting for a very long time and missed out on almost half a century of psychiatric progress. Yet it is a very real illness and, were it recognized adequately, would prove to be very much more common than we think. Many of its sufferers keep themselves to themselves, either not viewing themselves as ill or else being unwilling to accept a psychiatric formulation of their distress. Other individuals land in the hands of anyone but the psychiatrist, including police, lawyers, charismatic preachers, vermin control operators, dermatologists, infectious disease specialists and cosmetic surgeons and no doubt many more. This dispersal of cases into many other societal areas means that no one, least of all the mental health specialist, ever gets the whole picture. As we begin to grasp the larger aspects of the illness we start to get an impression of a very considerable impact on society at large. The somatic (hypochondriacal) subtype of delusional disorder may well impose a huge cost on health services as sufferers attend multiple doctors and demand wholly inappropriate investigations and treatments. Individuals with persecutory delusions may cause considerable disruption in their communities as well as running up against law enforcement agencies. Jealousy and erotomanic subtypes can lead to violence and even murder, sometimes even involving national and international figures as victims.

Then we enter into an area of pure speculation which is more than a little controversial. Some delusional disorder patients can remain highly functioning in society, either hiding their delusions very effectively or else channelling them into some quasi-acceptable expression. Some harmless cranks, some eccentric innovators, and some rather unbalanced community advocates may fall into this category and may even have a fairly useful function, acting as anti-establishment gadflies. But what about people who express their extreme and totally irremediable views and become part of a malignant belief system or an undesirable public movement? Some individuals who appear to be reasonable in most ways but who have a single, insistent theme which contradicts society's norms and which they persist in expressing against all debate or evidence must be suspected of having delusional beliefs; for example, respectable people with apparently normal lives who propagate virulent racial hatred and who cannot be convinced otherwise or persuaded to cease doing this. The end-point of this process, as suggested in Chapter 6, may be a figure like Hitler. There is no proof of this, but one would certainly suggest that some virulent antisemitics, like some recidivist sexual stalkers, have a delusional disorder and that it might be more possible to deal with them effectively if that were proven to be the case. Anyone can see the difficulties inherent in this proposition and the potential protests of civil rights advocates against the real danger of inappropriate psychiatric labelling of political dissidents. But if some of these dissidents are sick to the point of being an ever-present danger to society, and if our current law enforcement systems cannot influence their unbalanced beliefs, we may have to move to a different and more productive conceptualization of the problem they present, especially if that problem could be shown to be initiated by an illness.

Delusional disorder – making order out of chaos

Very often, cases of paranoia/delusional disorder have been recognized and labelled according to the content of their delusional system, hence de Clérambault's syndrome (erotomania), the Othello syndrome (jealousy), delusional parasitosis (somatic subtype), and so on. When we use superficial denominators such as these, then we invariably get very mixed bags of illnesses, so that a category of hypochondriacal delusional conditions could include cases of delusional disorder, schizophrenia, depressive illness with delusions, delirium, dementia and so on. In delusional disorder we recognize subtypes according to the delusional theme, but the illness itself has a number of other features (as described in Chapter 2) which give it a unique form and enable us to differentiate it from other psychiatric illnesses. It takes experience with a certain number of cases to appreciate that form and to be reasonably confident of the diagnosis. It is like reading a document in which one's name is mentioned: it seems to leap out of the text because we all have the 'shape' of our printed or written name engraved on our perceptions and it has a special significance. Similarly, the experienced clinician will be able to combine his or her theoretical knowledge of delusional disorder with his learned ability to recognize it in practice, and make an informed diagnosis. That demands a learning process and many mental health practitioners simply have not yet gone through that process, so they are not confident in recognition of delusional disorder.

When DSMIIIR revived the Kraepelinian description of paranoia and returned it to recognition as delusional disorder, it taught us a lesson which applies to other areas of psychiatric illness. It was an admission that, because of preconceptions and biases, an illness can be sidelined. Since the cases do not go away they will therefore be mis-labelled and, in the example of delusional disorder, this was usually as schizophrenia. If cases are mis-labelled they will be given the wrong treatments, and it will be impossible to carry out research on the illness because it is not separately conceptualised. This is not an isolated phenomenon and, in the past generations we have seen unipolar and bipolar mood disorders differentiated from each other, panic disorder separated from other types of anxiety disorder and obsessive–compulsive disorder upgraded from an uncommon to a common illness, to name but a few. We can only hope that our highly subjective diagnostic approaches in psychiatry will soon be backed up by a much more scientific methodology, as now seems increasingly likely, and also by an increasingly critical look at the loose concepts, constructs and terminology which are so often taken for granted in psychiatry (Schmidt, Tanner and Dent, 1996).

The world, and psychiatry within it, have changed enormously in the past 60 years and we are now all but divorced from the belief systems which prevailed in the psychiatry of the first third of the twentieth century. (A notable exception is Kraepelin's enduring classificatory schema for the major psychiatric disorders, and even that is now beginning to be challenged by the impact of new physiopathological discoveries.) Delusional disorder disappeared into limbo at a time of unsubstantiable theorising and therapeutic inertia in psychiatry: it reappeared in an era of very active treatment in the specialty as a whole and, by good fortune, it was shown to be treatable. Sadly, as mentioned in Chapter 13, some authors still go on repeating the dogma that it is untreatable, or denying that the treatments which have been described can be of any value. This is probably because, in all the changes occurring in psychiatry, delusional disorder has not yet made sufficient impact to create a memorable new impression or to challenge long-established ideas which no longer have relevance to new discoveries. It is hoped that the present volume will present a necessary challenge and a stimulus to think in contemporary terms.

The paranoid spectrum

Another important issue is at stake. When paranoia vanished, it did so in the company of other illnesses. Paraphrenia had a somewhat less secure footing than paranoia in the early part of the twentieth century, but it was still a widely utilized diagnosis. Even nowadays a small number of psychiatrists find it a useful concept. In this book and elsewhere the writer has tried to make as strong a case as possible for its resuscitation, and in Chapter 7 there is a suitably modernised clinical description *à la* DSMIV and ICD10. That is there for the use of any sufficiently motivated investigator.

Many psychiatrists seem to be aware of a gap in our diagnostic repertoire, especially between schizophrenia and delusional disorder. In discussing paraphrenia, the idea, which is quite venerable, was revived of a paranoid spectrum which would cover that gap and would include paraphrenia and (as originally proposed by Kraepelin) paranoid schizophrenia. In Chapter 8 the notion of a separate category of 'late' paraphrenia is challenged and it is proposed that this was simply paraphrenia arising for the first time in the elderly. It is also suggested that, since schizophrenia of late onset increasingly resembles paranoid schizophrenia as the patient gets older, differentiation between paraphrenia of first onset and schizophrenia of first onset in the extremely old may only be possible on neuroinvestigative, rather than on purely clinical, grounds.

Because we are increasingly directed in our diagnostic habits by official classificatory systems, many psychiatrists are unwilling to use diagnostic labels that are not sanctioned by ICD10 or DSMIV. These systems are influenced by biases, demands from local constituencies and, at times, by sheer ignorance of certain aspects of practice or of the literature. A favourite manoeuvre to avoid introducing a diagnosis that is at all controversial is to provide cover-all designations such as 'atypical' or 'not otherwise specified'. In this author's view, the term 'schizoaffective' really falls into this type of residual category, subsuming any illness which has a mixture of mood and schizophrenia-like symptoms and which cannot readily be placed elsewhere. If paraphrenia were an accepted diagnosis, many cases now called 'atypical', 'NOS' or 'schizoaffective' could more logically be re-designated. One cannot help thinking that, if delusional disorder had not declared its independence in 1987, it too would be consigned nowadays to these same meaningless, left-over categories, because at least it is now recognized that it is not schizophrenia.

In Chapter 9 there is strong promotion of the delusional misidentification syndromes (DMSs) as candidates for inclusion in an expanded group of delusional disorders. This has been done for two main reasons. In the first place its characteristics make it appear remarkably similar in many ways to the current description of paranoia/delusional disorder and, has been mentioned, there have been cases recorded in which characteristics of both illnesses coexist and overlap. Yet at present, DMS is not officially recognized by either of the major psychiatric diagnostic systems. Secondly, and more important than a purely taxonomic argument, is the fact that, in recent years, DMS has become associated with significant discoveries of relatively specific brain pathologies alongside its delusional phenomenology. This, from a psychiatric viewpoint, represents a breakthrough in methodology which could be applied to delusional disorder itself. If that occurred, we could rapidly break out of our old conceptual straitjacket and begin to study delusional disorder, and even delusions, in an objective and verifiable way.

Delusional disorder as an object of investigation

In Chapter 1 delusional disorder was presented as a potentially profitable object of study to help us gain *entrée* to understanding of psychotic disorders as a whole. It is a chronic but relatively stable illness, and it may well be the result of a very focal abnormality of brain function (similar to DMS). Because most of its sufferers refuse to see a psychiatrist or accept psychotropic medication, their brains are usually unaffected by such medication. Nevertheless, if they do accept treatment their illness can respond quite rapidly, thus allowing for studies of contrast between the pre-therapeutic state and drug-induced change. If DMS can be used as an analogy, it would also be possible to study parallel improvements in brain pathology and in clinical (i.e. delusional) manifestations, thereby giving some objective underpinning to the latter. Fortunately we are beginning to see the early stages of such investigations, although, as mentioned in Chapter 8, these are so far mostly in elderly patients who are likely to have a greater variety of brain changes due to organic factors than younger individuals with delusional disorder. It is hoped that more investigators will try to gather series of younger patients for investigation in the future.

'The delusional disorders'

Schizophrenia defies adequate investigation because it is such a large and incoherent grouping of different disorders lumped together as a result of superficial similarities. It is gradually breaking up and delusional disorder is 'the one that got away', thereby making it possible to treat and investigate it on its own.

If one argues for a paranoid spectrum, this is not to advocate lumping delusional disorder, paraphrenia, paranoid schizophrenia, and delusional misidentification syndromes together as one illness. Each is a discrete disorder but they have certain features in common and they appear to be interrelated with each other by lying on a kind of phenomenological continuum. It would improve our thinking about these conditions and make research on them simpler if it were officially recognized that they relate to each other much more closely than any of them relates to schizophrenia. This, in turn, would make it easier to study schizophrenia without the confounding presence of these other illnesses.

The future

It has recently been commented that eight-tenths of what we know about the brain's functions has been learned in the past decade, utilizing increasingly sophisticated electronic and computer-enhanced technologies. As these words are being written, delusional disorder has only been with us for that same decade and it has not had time to impress many practitioners with its presence or importance, or to find its way towards the laboratories.

That will change, and the change may well be rapid as it is realized how attractive it could be as a medium for studying the links between presumably circumscribed brain pathology and relatively specific psychiatric symptomatology. Quasi-philosophical speculation will give way to objective observation and perhaps the traditional psychopathology we now require to make our diagnosis of delusional disorder – especially delusion itself – will simply become the epiphenomena which point us towards the presence of illness, the illness to be defined thereafter by psychophysiological criteria.

For the present, this book should have raised its readers' level of consciousness about paranoia/delusional disorder in all its forms and with its many associated phenomena. It has attempted to re-interpret the illness and its treatment in a modern idiom and it has – realistically – presented the treatment of the illness in relatively optimistic terms. It has indicated what is outdated and should be abandoned and has emphasized what is most dependable in our current credo, and can point us most reliably to the future. It has stressed that greatly increased precision in diagnosis is possible even with our currently unsatisfactory criteria.

The topic is both fascinating and challenging. One can commend it as a fruitful area of research with a potential to further an investigator's career. Even more it can be commended as a clinical field where it is possible, with patience and care, to do a great deal for suffering patients who, because of their misguided ideas about the type of help they need, prove to be their own worst enemies in prolonging that suffering.

Reference

Schmidt, U., Tanner, M. and Dent, J.(1996). Evidence-based psychiatry: pride and prejudice. *Psychiat. Bull.* **20**: 705–707.

Recommended reading

Bhugra, D. and Munro, A. (Eds.) (1997). *Troublesome Disguises: Underdiagnosed Psychiatric Syndromes.* Oxford: Blackwell Science.

Cash, T.F. and Pruzinsky, T. (Eds.) (1990). *Body Images: Development, Deviance and Change.* New York: Guildford Press.

Garety, P.A. and Hemsley, D.R. (1994). *Delusions: Investigations into the Psychology of Delusional Reasoning.* Maudsley Monograph No. 36. Oxford: Oxford University Press.

Manschrek, T.C. (Ed.) (1992). Delusional disorders. *Psychiat. Ann.* **22**: 225–285.

Munro, A. (1982). *Delusional Hypochondriasis.* Clarke institute of Psychiatry Monograph No. 5. Toronto: Clarke Institute of Psychiatry.

Rix, K.J.B. and Snaith, R.P. (Eds.) (1988). The psychopathology of body image. *Br. J. Psychiat.* **153**: Supplement 2.

Sedler, M.J. (Ed.) (1995). Delusional disorders. *Psychiat. Clin. N. Am.* **18**: 199–425

Sharma, V.P. (1991). *Insane Jealousy*, Cleveland, Tennessee: Mind Publications.

Index